Stress Relief Urban Planning

Samaneh Jalilisadrabad • Mostafa Behzadfar
Khatereh Moghani Rahimi

Stress Relief Urban Planning

Springer

Samaneh Jalilisadrabad
School of Architecture &
Environmental Design
Iran University of Science &
Technology (IUST)
Tehran, Iran

Mostafa Behzadfar
School of Architecture &
Environmental Design
Iran University of Science &
Technology (IUST)
Tehran, Iran

Khatereh Moghani Rahimi
School of Architecture &
Environmental Design
Iran University of Science &
Technology (IUST)
Tehran, Iran

ISBN 978-981-99-4201-5 ISBN 978-981-99-4202-2 (eBook)
https://doi.org/10.1007/978-981-99-4202-2

This Springer imprint is published by the registered company Springer Nature Singapore Pte Ltd.
The registered company address is: 152 Beach Road, #21-01/04 Gateway East, Singapore 189721, Singapore

Foreword

The beginning of the industrial revolution in the nineteenth century and the changes and transformations that followed made towns restless and made people suffer from illnesses like depression, anxiety, stress, and other similar conditions. Stress is one of the most pervasive aspects of modern life, with many consequences for humans in terms of physical health, mental health, social issues, etc. Stress is a psychological problem and one of the most important fields of research in various sciences, which have received the attention of scientists from various fields, including doctors, psychologists, physiologists, biologists, and sociologists. Urban engineering, as a discipline addressing and studying all fields related to humans and their environment, must consider human health, especially mental health, and stress. By providing proper city planning, urban planning, as a specialized sub-field of this discipline, can help reduce stressful factors and their negative effects on citizens, resulting in improved mental health of citizens. To this end, this book tries to develop stress-relief urban planning using an interdisciplinary approach and take a step towards enhancing knowledge in this research field. The book *Stress Relief Urban Planning* is a comprehensive guide for urban planners who seek to reduce urban stress in the urban environment but lack proper training and texts. Also, by reading this book, urban designers will have a unified vision to reduce urban stress caused by the appearance of the city environment. Also, reading this book is highly recommended for city managers and policymakers. This book will aid urban psychologists, sociologists, architects, and social science scholars in better understanding the connection between their field and stress relief urban planning because it identifies urban policies that lessen urban stress and stressful urban factors. This book is written to be suitable for reading by general audiences and people from other professions and social strata. Reading this book is very useful for anyone who lives in the city or is under urban stress.

Contents

List of Figures

List of Tables

About the Authors

Samaneh Jalilisadrabad is an Assistant Professor in Regional and Urban Planning; Faculty Member of the School of Architecture and Environmental Design at Iran University of Science and Technology (IUST) since 2018, and Founder and Manager of Islamic Wisdom in Urban and Society Research Laboratory; Iran University of Science and Technology. She also currently serves as an editorial manager of the Armanshahr Architecture and Urban Design journal. She holds a PhD and MA in Regional and Urban Planning from the Iran University of Science and Technology, and a BA in Sociology from the University of Tehran. With his professional work, he has completed more than 16 projects in the field of Regional and Urban Planning and Urban sociology in the period of 2018–2023. On the other hand, in scientific-professional work, he teaches a variety of subjects including theory, methods, and techniques of Regional and Urban Planning, various workshops (especially regional and urban planning), research methods, and so on, especially at the masters and doctoral levels in IUST. She has published more than 60 papers in national and international journals. She has also presented papers at national and international conferences. Her major researches focus on urban sociology and urban planning.

Mostafa Behzadfar holds the positions of professor of urban design, a faculty member in the school of architecture and environmental design at the Iran University of Science and Technology, and dean of that school since 2016. He also founded and has been the manager of the university's Smart City Laboratory since 2013. He was born in 1956, graduated from Tehran University with a master's in urban planning in 1984, and Sydney University in Australia awarded him a doctorate (1997). He started his professional activity in 1977 (his student time). He also started his scientific-educational work as an assistant in the faculty of Fine Arts (1979–1980). With his professional work, he has completed more than 700 projects in the field of construction, architecture, and urban development (especially in urban design) from 1977 to 2021. On the other hand, in scientific-professional work, he teaches a variety of subjects including architectural design, theory of urban design, methods, and techniques of place-making basics, various workshops (especially urban design), research methods, and so on, especially at the master's and doctoral levels in different universities, mainly in Iran university of science and technology, as well as Shahid Beheshti, Tehran, and other universities. In line with scientific research activities, with hundreds of articles and more than 20 books, it has scientific-educational writings, especially books in the field of urban planning and design in its portfolio. From the executive point of view, he manages the school of architecture and environmental design projects and consulting engineers as well as the technical office of universities. Before his employment at the university, he held various responsibilities in the Ministry of Roads and Urban Development (Yazd Province Urban Land Organization) and the Yazd Governor's Office (Mehriz Municipality). In addition to his official work in the university, he worked as head of the department, vice chancellor, and dean of the school.

Khatereh Moghani Rahimi At Iran University of Science and Technology (IUST), Khatereh Moghani Rahimi works as a researcher in the Smart City study lab. She has a BA in urban planning from Lorestan University and an MA in urban planning from IUST. He has more than three articles published in some national journals. Additionally, she has delivered more than seven presentations at conferences held both domestically and abroad. Her major researches focus on urban psychology and urban planning.

Chapter 1
Introduction

Abstract Exposure to high stress and its resulting damages are critical factors enhancing the risk of mental disorders (Streit et al., Stress 17(4), 352–361, 2014). The stress induced by the modern urban lifestyle can be a ground for the development and prevalence of mental disorders (Kennedy and Adolphs, Nature 474(7352), 452–453, 2011; Wandersman and Nation, Am Psychol 53(6), 647–656, 1998). In addition to being a significant cause of physical and mental illness, urban stress also increases the rate of moral anomalies in the city, thereby reducing citizens' security. Moreover, it causes the loss of human capital in the city since high medical costs are imposed on citizens, and it reduces the quality of life and the level of satisfaction of citizens with the urban environment. Considering the stress difference in the world cities and its increase, urban planners, urban managers, and urban designers should urgently consider it an essential principle in their plans and designs to reduce its side effects.

In this chapter, materials such as: Background and aim, Benefits to the audience, Structure of this book are mentioned. Also, the content of each chapter of the book (Chap. 1: Introduction, Chap. 2: Explaining Related Concepts and Vocabulary and Identifying Their Connections, Chap. 3: Description of Urban Stressors, Chap. 4: Explaining Strategies to Reduce Urban Stress, Chap. 5: Identification of Urban Stress Measurement Methods, Chap. 6: Examining the Background and Global Experiences and Presenting Study Challenges and Gaps, Chap. 7: Presenting the Theoretical Framework of Stress Relief Urban Planning, Chap. 8: Conclusion) is described in the Structure of this book section.

Keywords Urban health · Urban mental health · Urban stress · Stress relief urban planning

S. Jalilisadrabad et al., *Stress Relief Urban Planning*,
https://doi.org/10.1007/978-981-99-4202-2_1

1.1 Background and Aim

Cities are growing quickly [1]. For the first time in 2007, more than 50% of the global populace lived in urban areas [2]. According to projections, by the year 2020, 70% of the world's population will live in urban areas, with Africa and Asia accounting for 90% of this increase [3]. Despite the advantages of cities over villages, living in urban regions has long been recognized as a risk factor for mental illness [4]. Urbanization has a significant negative effect on mental health and stress that is expected to get worse over the next [5]. Because it is a crucial aspect of public health and has a significant impact on people, communities, and the economy, mental health is a pressing problem [6]. Therefore, it is crucial to support it in order to enhance societal resilience and quality of life. Mental illness is now one of the major dangers to human health in 2020, according to the World Health Organization [7]. Mental illnesses affect one in five people worldwide and are responsible for 13% of the global disease burden [8, 9]. The World Psychiatric Association created the scientific section "urban mental health" to further research the relationship between urban life and mental health because of how important it is [10].

Exposure to high stress and its resulting damages are critical factors enhancing the risk of mental disorders [11]. The stress induced by the modern urban lifestyle can be a ground for the development and prevalence of mental disorders [12, 13]. In addition to being a significant cause of physical and mental illness, urban stress also increases the rate of moral anomalies in the city, thereby reducing citizens' security. Moreover, it causes the loss of human capital in the city since high medical costs are imposed on citizens, and it reduces the quality of life and the level of satisfaction of citizens with the urban environment. Considering the stress difference in the world cities and its increase, urban planners, urban managers, and urban designers should urgently consider it an essential principle in their plans and designs to reduce its side effects.

Although the expression of the relationship between urbanization and stress is the result of the study by Simmel [14], Prindle [15], Proshansky [16], Lazarus and Cohen [17], Baum et al. [18], Cohen et al. [19] and the need for a comprehensive operational framework to promote mental health was the main result of Christmas [20], demonstrated by Lederbogen et al. [21], Steinheuser et al. [22], Evans et al. [1], caused considerable attention to this issue. Given that many previous studies such as Burton [23], Jaffee et al. [24], Rishi and Khuntia [25], have examined urban stressors and studies such as Lin and Lai [26], Mukherjee and Agrawal [27] have examined models of stress in the urban environment. Separate studies same have explored the relationship between a particular indicator and urban stress, such as Haines et al. [28], Seth et al. [29], Freeman et al. [30], Li and Liu [31], Shannon et al. [32], Hernandez et al. [33] while there is no comprehensive study that includes all indicators.

In 2016, the term "neuro urbanism" was proposed for the first time as a solution to urban stress, which resulted in the "Nurourbanism Charter" in 2019 [34]. The interdisciplinary Society Neurourbanistics under the leadership of the Berlin

University Medical Center and consisting of neuroscientists, psychiatrists, psychologists, architects, urban planners, sociologists, geographers, and philosophers, published the "Neurourbanistic Charter" in 2019, which prioritized research and summarized the initial recommendations for action for psychologically healthier cities [35].

Numerous studies have examined the connection between urbanization and stress and its effective treatment using a variety of strategies, according to the study background. Even though not having proper urban planning is one factor that increases the amount of urban stress, there is no study describing and analyzing how stress can be relieved by urban planning. As a result, the proposed book aimed to describe stress relief urban planning. This book seeks to answer the following questions:

What is stress relief urban planning?
What use can this planning have?

Numerous studies have examined the connection between urbanization and stress and its effective treatment using a variety of strategies, according to the study background. Then they will have a comprehensive understanding of urban stressors and effective solutions, and they will get to know the experiences and background of research in this field. Then, the research challenges and gaps are clarified, and the stress relief urban planning framework is described.

1.2 Benefits to the Audience

The book *Stress Relief Urban Planning* is a comprehensive guide for urban planners who seek to reduce urban stress in the urban environment but lack proper training and texts. Also, by reading this book, urban designers will have a unified vision to reduce urban stress caused by the appearance of the city environment. Also, reading this book is highly recommended for city managers and policymakers. This book will aid urban psychologists, sociologists, architects, and social science scholars in better understanding the connection between their field and stress relief urban planning because it identifies urban policies that lessen urban stress and stressful urban factors. This book is written to be suitable for reading by general audiences and people from other professions and social strata. Reading this book is very useful for anyone who lives in the city or is under urban stress.

1.3 Structure of This Book

This book, first, explains basic concepts such as stress, urban stress, environmental stress, etc., and reviews relevant theoretical foundations. Then, it addresses the concept of stress relief urban planning, urban stress relief strategies, research

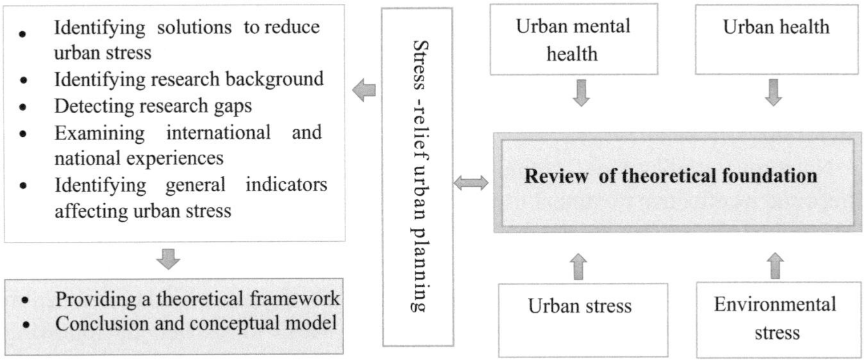

Fig. 1.1 The overall process of the book

background, research gaps, international and national experiences, and general indicators affecting urban stress. Finally, it provides a conceptual model and a theoretical framework for stress-relief urban planning by content analysis of previous studies and studying the relationships between the indicators. Figure 1.1 shows the overall process of this book and the next chapters are explained in the following.

1.3.1 Chapter 1: Introduction

This section presents the main problem and significance of compiling the book, its purpose, and a summary of the following chapters.

1.3.2 Chapter 2: Explaining Related Concepts and Vocabulary and Identifying Their Connections

This chapter explains concepts such as health, urban health, mental health, urban mental health, stress, and urban stress, then defines the relationship between these terms using the content analysis technique.

1.3.3 Chapter 3: Description of Urban Stressors

In this chapter, stress factors and their types are first described, then urban stress factors are identified from international studies and their classification. This chapter analyzes and categorizes urban stressors defined in international studies using categorical content analysis. Finally, each identified stressful factor has been explained.

1.3.4 Chapter 4: Explaining Strategies to Reduce Urban Stress

This chapter describes the solutions to reduce urban stress, such as: holding workshops to promote mental health, improving access to mental health services, improving the lighting of houses and urban spaces, improving the access and quality of green spaces, and compiling and implementing a comprehensive plan for mental health, and promoting urban design, promoting mental health, reducing time wastage and time pressure on citizens, promoting urban therapeutic gardening, controlling population density and building density, promoting urban resilience, promoting identity and sense of belonging to the city, revitalizing cultural and religious rituals, fostering social support and reducing deprivation, enhancing social activities of separation times, promoting local integration, increasing people's control over the environment, applying the principles of smart growth and new urbanism, not using outdated styles such as modern style, reducing economic deprivation, reducing pollution in urban environments, promoting justice, encouraging proper diet and reducing malnutrition, and fostering diversity in the urban environment and implementation of urban reform strategies.

1.3.5 Chapter 5: Identification of Urban Stress Measurement Methods

The techniques used to measure urban stress are described in this chapter, along with the benefits and drawbacks of doing so. The most effective way to measure urban stress is given in the chapter summary.

1.3.6 Chapter 6: Examining the Background and Global Experiences and Presenting Study Challenges and Gaps

This chapter consists of two sections: research background and global experiences. Study challenges and gaps are presented in the first section, which looks at the history of the study on urban mental health and urban stress. In the second section, global experiences related to urban mental health are explored, and issues and challenges are presented.

1.3.7 Chapter 7: Presenting the Theoretical Framework of Stress Relief Urban Planning

This chapter describes the concept of stress relief urban planning first. Then, according to the identified stressful factors, indicators have been identified, and relationships between them are defined using content analysis. Finally, the theoretical framework and conceptual model of this planning are presented.

1.3.8 *Chapter 8: Conclusion*

This section summarizes the previous chapters, presents conclusions, and recommends suggestions for future study.

References

1. Evans BE, van der Ende J, Greaves-Lord K, Huizink AC, Beijers R, de Weerth C. Urbanicity, hypothalamic-pituitary-adrenal axis functioning, and behavioral and emotional problems in children: a path analysis. BMC Psychol. 2020;8:12. https://doi.org/10.1186/s40359-019-0364-2.
2. Nnebue CC, Adinma ED, Queencallista N. Urbanization and health. Orient J Med. 2014;26:1–2.
3. Kirkbride JB, Keyes KM, Susser E. City living and psychotic disorders—implications of global heterogeneity for theory development. JAMA Psychiatry. 2018;75:1211–2. https://doi.org/10.1001/jamapsychiatry.2018.2640.
4. Adli M. Urban stress and mental health. Cities, Health and Well-Being, Hong Kong; 2011.
5. Evans BE, Huizink AC, Greaves-Lord K, Tulen JHM, Roelofs K, van der Ende J, Santana GL. Urbanicity, biological stress system functioning and mental health in adolescents. PLoS One. 2020;15(3):e0228659. https://doi.org/10.1371/journal.pone.0228659.
6. Lloyd S, Kelly R, Kimberly G, Joshua R. Challenges of urban mental health disaster planning. J Aggress Maltreat Trauma. 2005;10(3):695–706. https://doi.org/10.1300/J146v10n03_03.
7. Larcombe E, Logan P, Horwitz A. High-rise apartments and urban mental health—historical and contemporary views. Challenges. 2019;10(2):34. https://doi.org/10.3390/challe10020034.
8. Helbich M. Toward dynamic urban environmental exposure assessments in mental health research. Environ Res. 2018;161:129–35. https://doi.org/10.1016/j.envres.2017.11.006.
9. Joshua CF, Freeman C, Bazargan-Hejazi S. Environmental interventions for physical and mental health: challenges and opportunities for greater Los Angeles. Int J Environ Res Public Health. 2019;16(12):2180. https://doi.org/10.3390/ijerph16122180.
10. Caracci G. General concepts of the relationship between urban areas and mental health. Curr Opin Psychiatry. 2008;21(4):385–90. https://doi.org/10.1097/yco.0b013e328303e198.
11. Streit F, Haddad L, Paul T, Frank J, Schäfer A, Nikitopoulos J, et al. A functional variant in the neuropeptide S receptor 1 gene moderates the influence of urban upbringing on stress processing in the amygdala. Stress. 2014;17(4):352–61. https://doi.org/10.3109/10253890.2014.921903.
12. Kennedy DP, Adolphs R. Social neuroscience: stress and the city. Nature. 2011;474(7352):452–3. https://doi.org/10.1038/474452a.
13. Wandersman A, Nation M. Urban neighborhoods and mental health. Psychological contributions to understanding toxicity, resilience, and interventions. Am Psychol. 1998;53(6):647–56.
14. Simmel J. The metropolis and mental life. Section 7 of the people, place, and space reader, 1903, p. 223–6.
15. Prindle RA. Health aspects of the urban environment. Public Health Rep (1896–1970). 1968;83(7):617–21. https://doi.org/10.2307/4593367.
16. Proshansky HM. Urban stress. Experiments on noise and social stressors. David C. Glass and Jerome E. Singer. Academic Press, New York, 1972. xiv, 182 pp., illus. $8.75. Social Psychology. Science. 178(4067):1275A. https://doi.org/10.1126/science.178.4067.1275a.
17. Lazarus RS, Cohen JB. Environmental stress. Hum Behav Environ. 1977;1977:89–127. https://doi.org/10.1007/978-1-4684-0808-9_3.
18. Baum AS, Jerome EB, Carlene S. Stress and the environment. Soc Issues. 1981;37(1):4–35. https://doi.org/10.1111/j.1540-4560.1981.tb01056.x.

19. Cohen S, Evans GW, Stokols D, Krantz DS. Environmental stress and cognitive performance. In: Cohen S, Evans GW, Stokols D, Krantz DS, editors. Behaviour, health, and environmental stress. Berlin: Springer; 1986. p. 143–83.
20. Christmas JJ. Psychological stresses of urban living: new direction for mental health services in the inner city. J Natl Med Assoc. 1973;65(6):483–6, passim.
21. Lederbogen F, Kirsch P, Haddad L, Streit F, Tost H, Schuch P, et al. City living and urban upbringing affect neural social stress processing in humans. Nature. 2011;474:498–501.
22. Steinheuser V, Ackermann K, Pia A, Lars S. Stress and the city. Psychosom Med. 2014;76(9):678–85. https://doi.org/10.1097/PSY.0000000000000113.
23. Burton I. Factors in urban stress. J Sociol Soc Welf. 1990;17(1):Article 5.
24. Jaffee KD, Liu GC, Canty-Mitchell J, Qi RA, Austin J, Swigonski N. Race, urban community stressors, and behavioral and emotional problems of children with special health care needs. Psychiatr Serv. 2005;56(1):63–9. https://doi.org/10.1176/appi.ps.56.1.63.
25. Rishi P, Khuntia G. Urban environmental stress and behavioral adaptation in Bhopal City of India. Urban Stud Res. 2012;2012:1–9. https://doi.org/10.1155/2012/635061.
26. Lin N, Lai G. Urban stress in China. Soc Sci Med. 1995;41(8):1131–45. https://doi.org/10.1016/0277-9536(94)00426-t.
27. Mukherjee A, Agrawal M. The influence of urban stress factors on responses of ground cover vegetation. Environ Sci Pollut Res. 2018;25:36194–206. https://doi.org/10.1007/s11356-018-3437-5.
28. Haines MM, Stansfeld SA, Job RFS, Berglund B, Head J. Chronic aircraft noise exposure, stress responses, mental health and cognitive performance in school children. Psychol Med. 2001;31(2):265–77. https://doi.org/10.1017/S0033291701003282.
29. Seth P, Murray CC, Braxton ND, DiClemente RJ. The concrete jungle: city stress and substance abuse among young adult African American men. J Urban Health. 2012;90(2):307–13. https://doi.org/10.1007/s11524-012-9716-4.
30. Freeman D, Emsley R, Dunn G, Fowler D, Bebbington P, Kuipers E, et al. The stress of the street for patients with persecutory delusions: a test of the symptomatic and psychological effects of going outside into a busy urban area. Schizophr Bull. 2015;41(4):971–9. https://doi.org/10.1093/schbul/sbu173.
31. Li J, Liu Z. Housing stress and mental health of migrant populations in urban China. Cities. 2018;81:172–9. https://doi.org/10.1016/j.cities.2018.04.006.
32. Shannon MM, Clougherty JE, McCarthy C, Elovitz MA, Nguemeni Tiako MJ, Melly SJ, et al. Neighborhood violent crime and perceived stress in pregnancy. Int J Environ Res Public Health. 2020;17(15):5585. https://doi.org/10.3390/ijerph17155585.
33. Hernandez DC, Daundasekara SS, Zvolensky MJ, Reitzel LR, Maria DS, Alexander AC, et al. Urban stress indirectly influences psychological symptoms through its association with distress tolerance and perceived social support among adults experiencing homelessness. Int J Environ Res Public Health. 2020;17(15):5301. https://doi.org/10.3390/ijerph17155301.
34. Adli M, Berger M, Brakemeier E-L, Engel L, Fingerhut J, Hehl R, et al. Neurourbanistik – ein methodischer Schulterschluss zwischen Stadtplanung und Neurowissenschaften. Die Psychiatrie. 2016;13:70–8.
35. Adli M, Schondorf J. Macht uns die Stadt krank. Wirkung von Stadtstress auf Emotionen, Verhalten und psychische Gesundheit; Does the city make us ill? The effect of urban stress on emotions, behavior, and mental health. Bundesgesundheitsbl. 2020;63:979–86. https://doi.org/10.1007/s00103-020-03185-w.

Chapter 2
Explaining Related Concepts and Vocabulary and Identifying Their Connections

Abstract In this chapter, concepts such as health, mental health, urban health, stress, environmental stress, and urban stress are fully described. Then, the relationships between these concepts and urban stress are identified through content analysis using MAXQDA software. Stress is a social pollutant, an unpleasant emotional state, an unspecific physiological and psychological response to perceived real and imagined threats and stress factors (environmental, social, and behavioral stimuli) to physical, mental, or social integrity, a mechanism preparing us for any reaction (biochemical, physiological, and behavioral response), and also making us evolve and adapt more to the environment. What it causes and what its effects are not always clear. It can be acute (appears suddenly through an unpredictable threat), or chronic (resulting from exposure to repeated threats). Although it is not harmful in general, exposure to chronic stress endangers our physical, mental, emotional, spiritual, and social health. It is an acute threat to the homeostasis (steady state) of an organism, which helps its physical and mental well-being. In fact, the nervous system alerts the body by increasing the heart rates and releasing some hormones (adrenaline and cortisol) and the body quickly turns to maximize its power. This automatic process is known as the "fight-or-flight" reaction or the "stress response." Urban stress is actually the cumulative stress caused by the experience of living in unfavorable conditions of the urban environment and a general term related to the relationship between the urban environment and its impact on human mental health and a reaction to some threats perceived by undesirable urban events such as pollution, high population, extreme temperature, crowding, noise, destroyed landscape, excessive accumulation of solid waste, waste of time in commuting, etc., and if these conditions are beyond the urbanite's tolerance, he will experience urban stress. The city both directly influences mental health and causes stress through social, economic, physical, environmental, housing, transportation, and individual stressors, and this stress reduces mental health. Of course, the city also influences mental health through the reduction of general or physical health, because the areas of health and mental health are largely interdependent. Mental health also affects the city both directly and through stress and public health. As a result, urban stress and physical health can mediate the effects of urbanization on mental health and the

S. Jalilisadrabad et al., *Stress Relief Urban Planning*,
https://doi.org/10.1007/978-981-99-4202-2_2

effects of mental health on the city. A better understanding of this relationship and the effect of mediators and trying to reduce the negative effects of cities on mental health will greatly help to best take advantage of urban life.

Keywords Urban health · Urban mental health · Environmental stress · Urban stress

2.1 Introduction

In this chapter, concepts such as health, mental health, urban health, stress, environmental stress, and urban stress are fully described. Then, the relationships between these concepts and urban stress are identified through content analysis using MAXQDA software.

2.2 Health

In 1986, the Ottawa Charter for Health Promotion was created. Next, this idea was repeated and expanded upon at the fourth international meeting on health promotion, which took place in Jakarta in 1997. According to the Jakarta Declaration, having good health is a fundamental human right and is essential to both societal and economic progress [1]. The definition of health is "a person's capacity to adjust and manage oneself in the face of physical, mental, and social challenges" [2]. Although there have been various definitions of health presented, the World Health Organization's preamble of its constitution contains the following definition, which is the most generally accepted health is described as a condition of total physical, mental, and social well-being, not just the absence of disease or infirmity, as well as the capacity to lead an economically and socially productive existence [2].

Ill health can result from individual conditions and choices (such as income), physical environment (such as housing, health facilities, and other services) [3], and social environment (such as norms, social networks, and stressors) [4].

Stress-related behavioral, lifestyle, socioeconomic, and environmental variables contribute to health issues. Health is strongly influenced by behavioral and socioeconomic factors. Health is influenced by environmental variables both directly and indirectly through socioeconomic and behavioural factors. There are feedback consequences in every situation. Numerous social, behavioral, and environmental factors may affect health, but their exact effects are unknown. Additionally, the potential synergistic impacts of various variables on one another are not fully understood [5].

2.3 Health and Urbanization

Due to rising birth rates and declining mortality, the global population is growing. This growth is more pronounced in the urban population and less developed nations due to problems like rural-urban migration and the conversion of rural settlements into urban ones. Cities are developing incredibly quickly, particularly in Southwest Asia and Northeast Africa [6]. For the first time in 2007, more people lived in cities than in rural areas, and this proportion is steadily increasing. They develop into a culture that is increasingly urban and urbanist [7]. Figure 2.1 illustrates that by 2025, 70% of the world's population is anticipated to live in cities, with 90% of this increase taking place in Africa and Asia [8, 9]. Due to the world's increasing urbanization, more and more people are facing risk factors brought on by the urban social and physical environments (such as poverty and air pollution) as well as rising stress levels and mental health disorders. Cities, on the other hand, offer greater access to employment, education, and healthcare. To strike a balance between these two issues, it is necessary to comprehend how urban living and health interact [10]. The impact of cities and urbanization on people's physical and mental well-being highlighted the need for planned urbanisation to mitigate these effects. Unfortunately, there are no official recommendations for giving cities healthier and more organised urbanisation [11].

Human health and his living environment are connected intricately. Also, the number of people and how they live through the use of natural resources and waste production influences the environment, and the environment, in turn, can influence human health through effects such as poor housing, poor sanitation, etc. [7]. In fact, poor physical characteristics of urban environments negatively affect public health [12]. This clarifies the significance of urban health as an international issue.

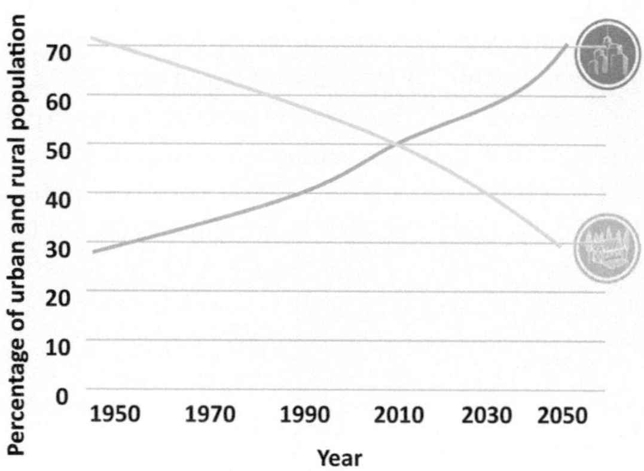

Fig. 2.1 Development of the global population in urban and rural areas by 2050 [8]

2.4 Urban Health

The study of urban characteristics, such as the elements of the social and physical environment, urban infrastructure, and resources, which can have an impact on health and illness in an urban setting, is referred to as urban health. Urban health research calls for an interdisciplinary approach and employs a variety of quantitative and qualitative techniques [13]. Numerous variables that have an impact on people's living conditions and the relationships between them are important to urban health. To fully comprehend urban health, it is necessary to consider behavioral, biological, cultural, economic, social, physical, and political factors [14].

It has become more challenging for cities to safeguard the health of all citizens as a result of migration patterns, shifts in the global economy, rising income inequality, etc. [1]. Numerous communicable and non-communicable diseases are listed as adverse effects of cities by the United Nations, and studies have shown that urbanisation increases the risk of diseases like diabetes, asthma, hypertension, metabolic syndrome, hearing disorders, sleep disorders, stress-related disorders, cognitive disorders [15]. Urban health cannot be completely discussed without mentioning the links between urban health and climate change. Cities are one of the main factors of climate change, and the changing climate change affects the health of citizens directly and indirectly [16]. Therefore, the city environment influences all aspects of health [17]. Also, this environment often has the human, financial, and social capital, the right employment of which should be considered to promote health [1].

Nowadays, protecting urban health has become a big challenge, especially in developing countries [18]. In this regard, the World Health Organization (WHO) conceived the Healthy Cities Initiative (HCI) in 1986 as a means to legitimize, foster, and support community empowerment [19]. Urban health poses risks to many various industries, including those in the fields of health, the environment, housing, energy, transportation, and urban planning, among others. To recognise the effects of urbanisation on both the global and personal levels on our collective health, WHO has selected the 2010 World Health Day theme of "Urbanization and Health." It aims to bring this issue to the attention of the world and to engage governments, businesses, and civil society in a cooperative effort to place health at the centre of urban policy [7]. In order to understand urban health more fully, it is therefore essential to study the dynamic nature of cities, the features of the context, and to closely monitor contextual changes influencing urban health [17].

2.5 Mental Health

Mental health is a very important issue considering its role as an essential component of public health [20]. It has profound impacts on individuals, societies, and the economy [20], and its promotion is required to raise the quality of life and resilience of society. In 2020, mental health disorders are expected to rank among the top risks to people's health, according to the World Health Organization. Due to the negative effects of stress, depression, and anxiety on people's ability to work efficiently, this problem also affects economic prosperity [21]. Nearly one in five adults in the world suffer from mental illness [22]. Also, according to the World Health Organization's mental health report (2003), mental disorders account for 13% of the global burden of diseases, while only 2% of the total health budgets of governments have been assigned to this issue. This disparity in policy and investment is associated with current limitations in technology, lack of data, and immaturity of awareness regarding mental illness, as compared to physical illness [23].

The disciplines of "health" and "mental health" are distinguished from each other in many ways, but they should not be considered separate from each other. Without mental health, there can be no physical health, and bodily illnesses also have an impact on mental health [20]. Experts continue to disagree on the exact definitions of "mental health" and "mental illness." Many socially unacceptable behaviors, or social pathologies, are mentioned by some researchers, including alcoholism, substance addiction, excessive medication use, sexual assault, domestic violence offenses, etc. as symptoms of mental illness, and express the relationship between these issues in the definition of mental health [5]. In fact, different studies can define, use, and measure mental health in significantly different ways [24]. Different definitions of mental health have been provided. The present research considers the definition given by Scully [25]. Some definitions of mental health are as follows:

- The ability to individually and collectively adjust to an environment and maintain homeostatic equilibrium in life, despite a changing environment, is what is meant by the term "mental health," which is basically a measure of resilience. However, a lot of data indicates that the modern environment is eroding resilience [21].
- Mental health is a widely used concept in social sciences. However, ambiguous definitions of it have been provided, which refer to psychological and emotional well-being [24].
- A person who is in good mental health is aware of his or her abilities, able to handle everyday stresses, able to work effectively and efficiently, and able to give

back to the community. Psychological well-being (self-acceptance, personal growth, optimism, hopefulness, purpose in life, control over one's environment, spirituality, self-direction, and positive relationships), social well-being (social acceptance, belief in the potential of people and society as a whole, presence of social determinants of mental health such as adequate housing, safe neighborhoods, equitable jobs and wages), and emotional well-being (life satisfaction, happiness, and peace of mind) are all components of well-being. The ability to learn, express, and manage a wide range of positive and negative emotions, maintain positive relationships with others, and deal with and manage change and uncertainty are all signs of good mental health. Good mental health is not just the absence of diagnosable mental problems [25].

- Mental health can be considered freedom from and the absence of mental illness. It can also be defined as well-being or life satisfaction [26].

2.6 Urbanization and Mental Health

Larger groups of people, and later cities, have always been viewed as safe havens away from the perils of living in remote locations as well as places where one can learn new skills and start a new existence. Because of the ongoing migration of people from rural to urban areas, these beliefs continue to persist [27]. Urbanization is a dynamic outcome of the complex interactions between population (size, density, and homogeneity), space-geography (location, climate, and land), historical, cultural, economic, and political forces for the creation of an environment and community that is psychologically and socially compatible [28].

Population health has long been a concern for cities. Because cities now house more than half of the world's population, creating a healthy urban environment is a top concern for policymakers. Since mood disorders and anxiety are more common in urban residents, urban living has an impact on mental health [29]. Living in an urban setting has long been recognised as a risk factor for mental illness, despite the fact that cities offer more and better infrastructure, socioeconomic conditions, nutrition, and healthcare facilities than rural areas [30]. Numerous studies have revealed that the connection between the urban environment and psychological issues is stronger over time and is more pronounced in young people than in older people [31]. Given that the urban population is expected to grow over the next few decades and that urbanisation has a significant negative effect on mental health [28]. Some researchers refer to this adverse effect as the "urbanization impact" because they believe it to be very significant [32]. However, studies on neighbourhood environments and population health have primarily paid attention to physical health, with less emphasis on mental health. Numerous studies have looked into the connection between neighbourhoods' social environments and mental health. But there are a lot fewer studies looking at possible connections between the built world and mental health [33]. When promoting urban mental health, it is helpful to concentrate on those aspects of the metropolitan environment that are most conducive to mental health [28]. The significance of creating urban planning based on mental health is made clear by this problem. Several research that looked into the connection between urbanisation and mental health are listed in Table 2.1.

According to Table 2.1, numerous studies in developed nations around the world, particularly in Europe and the United States, have linked urban life to a higher risk of mental health issues than rural life and have linked the rapid growth of cities to the higher risk of mental health issues. There are, of course, outliers. According to a New Zealand survey, rural residents' mental health is worse than that of city dwellers [62]. Urban life was found to not be associated with experiences of psychosis or psychotic disorder in another study on the relationship between urbanisation and psychosis in low- and middle-income countries. This finding conflicts with theoretical literature and the current divergence, suggesting that the relationship between urbanisation and psychosis may be specific to industrialised nations rather than being a global phenomenon. Of course, more research is required [64].

The use of stress-relieving medications was identified as an inappropriate indicator for measuring stress in areas due to the effectiveness of other factors such as people's income, access to health services, etc. in a study in New Zealand, and it was identified that there are mental health-reducing factors in the cities of

Table 2.1 Studies carried out on the impact of urbanization on mental health

	Research name	Authors	Year	Country	Impact	Reference
America	Rural–urban differences in the prevalence of major depression and associated impairment	Wang	2004	Canada	–	[34]
	Rural residence is not a risk factor for frequent mental distress: a behavioral risk factor surveillance survey	Rohrer et al.	2005	USA	–	[35]
	Schizophrenia and Urbanicity: A Major Environmental Influence—Conditional on Genetic Risk Schizophrenia and Urbanicity: A Major Environmental Influence—Conditional on Genetic Risk	Krabbendam and van Os	2005	USA, UK	–	[31]
	Correlates of Urban Stress and Mental Health: The Impact of Social Context on Resilience	Miller and Phillips	2005	USA	–	[27]
	Urban Mental Health: An International Survey	Caracci	2006	USA	–	[36]

(continued)

Table 2.1 (continued)

	Research name	Authors	Year	Country	Impact	Reference
Europe	Schizophrenia and city life	Lewis et al.	1992	Sweden	–	[37]
	Are cities bad for your mental health?	Lewis and Booth	1994	UK	–	[38]
	Urbanization and psychosis: a study of 1942–1978 birth cohorts in The Netherlands	Marcelis et al.	1998	Netherlands	–	[39]
	Urban–rural mental health differences in Great Britain: findings from the National Morbidity Survey	Paykel et al.	2000	UK	–	[40]
	Regional differences in schizophrenia incidence in Denmark	Schelin et al.	2000	Denmark	–	[41]
	Depressive disorders in Europe: Prevalence figures from the ODIN study	Ayuso-Mateos et al.	2001	Finland, Great Britain, Ireland, Norway	–	[42]
	Evidence of a Dose-Response Relationship Between Urbanicity During Upbringing and Schizophrenia Risk	Pedersen	2001	Denmark	–	[43]
	Comparison of the incidence of schizophrenia in rural Dumfries and Galloway and urban Camberwell	Allardyce et al.	2001	Scotland	–	[44]
	Association between psychotic disorder and urban place of birth is not mediated by obstetric complications or childhood socio-economic position: a cohort study	Harrison et al.	2003	Sweden	–	[45]
	Confirmation of Synergy Between Urbanicity and Familial Liability in the Causation of Psychosis	van Os et al.	2004	Denmark	–	[46]
	Urbanisation and incidence of psychosis and depression: Follow-up study of 4.4 million women and men in Sweden	Sundquist et al.	2004	Sweden	–	[47]

Table 2.1 (continued)

Research name	Authors	Year	Country	Impact	Reference
A European Approach to Rural—Urban Differences in Mental Health: The ESEMeD 2000 Comparative Study	Kovess-Masfety et al.	2005	Belgium, France, Germany, Italy, Holland, Spain	–	[48]
Rural/non-rural differences in rates of common mental disorders in Britain: Prospective multilevel cohort study	Weich et al.	2006	UK	–	[49]
Are the Cause(s) Responsible for Urban-Rural Differences in Schizophrenia Risk Rooted in Families or in Individuals?	Pedersen and Mortensen	2006	Denmark	–	[50]
Is the prevalence of psychiatric disorders associated with urbanization?	Peen et al.	2007	Netherlands	–	[51]
Psychiatric disorders and urbanization in Germany	Dekker et al.	2008	Germany	–	[52]
Urbanicity, social adversity and psychosis	Heinz et al.	2013	UK	–	[53]
Brain Structure Correlates of Urban Upbringing, an Environmental Risk Factor for Schizophrenia	Haddad et al.	2015	Germany	–	[54]
Urban-rural differences in incidence rates of psychiatric disorders in Denmark	Vassos et al.	2016	Denmark	–	[55]
A tool to predict perceived urban stress in open public spaces	Knöll et al.	2017	Germany	–	[56]
IQ, the Urban Environment, and Their Impact on Future Schizophrenia Risk in Men	Toulopoulou et al.	2017	Denmark	–	[57]
Cities and mental health	Gruebner et al.	2017	Germany	–	[10]
Sociology, biology and mechanisms in urban mental health	Manning	2018	UK	–	[58]

(continued)

Table 2.1 (continued)

	Research name	Authors	Year	Country	Impact	Reference
	Urbanicity, hypothalamic-pituitary-adrenal axis functioning, and behavioral and emotional problems in children: a path analysis	Evans et al.	2020a	Netherlands	–	[6]
Asia	Psychiatric Epidemiology in Korea	Lee et al.	1990	North Korea	–	[59]
	Urban stress and mental health	Adli	2011	China	–	[30]
	Depression, Anxiety, and Stress Among Urban and Rural Police Officers	Waqar	2019	Pakistan	–	[60]
	URBANICITY AND PSYCHOSIS IN A CHINESE UNDERGRADUATE POPULATION: PRELIMINARY FINDINGS	Coid et al.	2020	China	–	[61]
Australia	Rural-Urban Differences in the Use of Stress-Alleviative Drugs	Webb and Collette	1977	New Zealand	+	[62]
	A systematic review of the incidence of schizophrenia: the distribution of rates and the influence of sex, urbanicity, migrant status and methodology	McGrath et al.	2004	Saint Lucia	–	[63]
Other	Association of Urbanicity With Psychosis in Low- and Middle-Income Countries	DeVylder et al.	2018	–	+	[64]
	The current status of urban-rural differences in psychiatric disorders	Peen et al.	2010	–	–	[65]

non-industrialized countries such as Kabul, known as one of the most stressful cities. However, since many studies emphasized the poor mental health of urbanites, it is important to note that these factors are present in urban areas as. Additionally, there is a notable difference between urban and rural areas in terms of mental disorders, mood disorders, and anxiety disorders, according to Peen et al. [65] meta-analysis of the nations of Belgium, the United States, Germany, Spain, South Korea, Australia, the Netherlands, France, Italy, the United Kingdom, and Norway [65]. People with a genetic risk of mental health problems also tend to live in dense urban areas [66] in the hopes of better healthcare or to avoid the stigma of mental illness in rural areas. Living in urban environments is associated with different levels of stress and a greater risk of mental health problems [8, 67]. Due to selective migration, or the propensity of vulnerable individuals to migrate to urban regions, urbanisation may therefore have an impact on mental health [68]. However, urban living is also thought to be a separate risk factor for mental health issues [31]. Urbanization and psychological issues like depression, however, have a complicated connection that is likely mediated and moderated by a variety of other variables [69]. Urbanization is raising concerns about mental disorders around the globe, but developing nations like China, Iran, and India are less aware of this problem [70]. Sadly, there are currently no recognised international standards for preventing mental health issues linked to rapid urbanisation in these nations [11]. In higher-income cities that are rapidly developing Western values and societies, mental disorders are more common. These conditions place a heavy financial burden on municipal budgets [36]. A simple 20% decline in the prevalence of urban mental illness could result in annual savings of about $250 billion [71]. Of course, the costs of mental disorders go far beyond direct expenses and also include things like a higher likelihood of dropping out of school early, a lower chance of finding a job that is appropriate for one's skills, a lower quality of life, etc. [71].

According to the World Health Organisation, 4 out of 10 nations lack a mental health strategy, and in a third of the 181 nations looked at, there was no budget designated for mental health. It is challenging to systematically address the mental health requirements of urbanites because there are no mental health policies in place [36]. In fact, a deeper understanding of the connection between urbanisation and mental health issues may aid in the development of coping mechanisms and a better design for future cities that are more in line with human requirements [72]. The World Psychiatric Association has created a scientific department of urban mental health to further research the relationship between urban life and mental health because of its importance [73].

In this respect, it is important to encourage research studies and detailed guidelines to assist decision-makers and urban planners in enhancing mental health in cities. The world should also implement some measures to prevent and lessen mental illness in urban areas. Cities have grown in number as a result of rapid industrialization and globalisation, and foreign health policies need to take these new challenges into account [74]. A summary of this section's results is shown in Fig. 2.2.

Living in cities has numerous advantages over living in villages, including better access to education, services, and jobs, which are introduced as "advantages of urbanization" [71]. Stating that cities have negative effects on mental health doesn't imply anti-urbanism[1] or the false image that Park and his students had of the cities

[1] After the publication of Lucia Perry White and Morton White's book "The Intellectual Versus the City" in 1962, anti-urbanism and urbanism were noticed in America, and the peak of this approach can be seen in the works of John Dewey and Robert Park [75].

Urbanization is a global and growing phenomenon with many consequences on mental health.

The greatest increase in urbanization is occurring in developing countries, while they pay little attention to the issue of mental health.

In many developing or developed countries, government programs have allocated little funds to the issue of mental health.

Most of the relevant scientific studies on urban mental health have been conducted in developed countries and their results cannot be applied to low-income and middle-income countries because urbanization has different characteristics and consequences in different places.

In this regard, research studies and specific guidelines should be encouraged to help policymakers and urban designers to improve mental health in cities.

Some strategies to prevent and reduce mental illness in urban settings should also be adopted globally

There is no politically and professionally agreed international guidelines for appropriate urban planning of mental health services.

Fig. 2.2 Significant points concerning the relationship between urbanization and mental health [74]

[76]. Rather, this discussion aims to improve cities and reduce the negative effects of cities on mental health.

2.7 Stress

Hans Selye, known as the "father of stress," was the first to use the word "stress." He understood that individuals with vague symptoms react to outside stimuli [77]. Although the idea of stress was present in the late nineteenth century, it wasn't until after World War II that it became generally accepted in Britain. At first, it was used to explain the rise in stomach diseases like ulcers [78]. Georg Simmel, a German sociologist, first suggested this term in his scientific writings in 1903, and it has a long history [79]. There are numerous ways to define tension, some of which are provided below:

- Stress is an unspecific physiological and psychological response to perceived threats to physical, psychological, or social integrity. It is a mechanism preparing us for any reaction and also makes us evolve and adapt more to the environment.

Although it is not harmful in general, exposure to chronic stress endangers our health [4].
- Stress is an unpleasant emotional state experienced by people when they perceive a situation as unsafe or threatening to their well-being [29].
- Stress is a physical or mental stimulus that threatens a person [58].
- The concept of stress means environmental demands requiring adaptive responses from the individual. It is an environmental stimulus causing an individual to respond to it [16].
- Stress is a relationship between the individual and the environment, and the person appraises it as taxing or exceeding his resources and endangering his well-being [80].
- Stress is a function of the environment, and social and behavioral factors, although its cause and effect are not always clear [5].
- The concept of stress has been developed to describe environmental characteristics causing physical or psychological discomfort [81].
- Stress is a natural biological and emotional response to life events. It causes certain biochemical, physiological, and behavioral changes in a person. Stress can be acute (emerging suddenly through an unpredictable threat), or chronic (caused by exposure to repeated threats) [82].
- Stress is an acute threat to the homeostasis (steady state) of an organism. It contributes to physical and mental well-being, and sensitivity to it is a reflection of complex individual, social, social, and environmental factors. Humans can easily adapt to acute stress, but chronic stress negatively reduces performance and causes a wide range of mental illnesses, including schizophrenia, depression, and anxiety [21].
- Stress is a process in which events or environmental forces, called stressors, threaten an organism and the organism responds to this threat [83].
- Stress is defined as the body's unspecific response to threats due to internal and external factors [84].
- Stress is the way the human body responds to any real or unreal demand or threat and is a way the human body defends when facing danger. The nervous system alerts the body by increasing the heart rate and releasing some hormones (adrenaline and cortisol) and the body quickly turns to maximize its power. This automatic process is known as the "fight-or-flight" reaction or the "stress response." Thus, stress is not bad in all cases. However, if it becomes chronic stress, it would have significant negative effects on various dimensions (physical, mental, emotional, spiritual, and social) of human health [84].
- Psychological stress is conceptualized as a "social pollutant" that influences human health acutely and chronically and may disrupt biological systems through inflammatory processes. It can also affect humans' psychological and physiological performance and behavior [85].

According to the definitions presented above, a comprehensive definition of stress is as follows:

Stress is a social pollutant, an unpleasant emotional state, an irrational physiological and psychological reaction to perceived real and imagined threats and stress factors (environmental, social, and behavioural stimuli) to physical, mental, or social integrity, a mechanism that gets us ready for any reaction (biochemical, physiological, and behavioural response), as well as one that helps us evolve and adapt to our surroundings more. It's not always obvious what it causes or what its effects are. It can be acute (appearing abruptly as a result of an unforeseen threat) or chronic. (resulting from exposure to repeated threats). Even though it generally has no negative effects, long-term stress exposure poses a threat to our physical, mental, emotional, spiritual, and societal well-being. An organism's homeostasis, which promotes its physical and mental wellbeing and keeps it in a steady condition, is gravely threatened by this. The body responds rapidly to the nervous system's alarm by speeding up heart rates and releasing hormones (cortisol and adrenaline). The "fight-or-flight" reflex, also referred to as the "stress response," is this automatic process.

2.8 Environmental Stress

Both internal and external factors can cause stress. The ability of the human body to respond to external stress is determined by internal factors, whilst external factors are connected to the local built and natural environments. Stress is a constant process in which a person's perception of stimuli from their surroundings through many senses serves as the foundation for physical or intangible reactions [84]. Dealing with the local natural and manmade environment is thus one of the key variables determining human mental health [86]. Human behaviour depends on the individual, the environment, and how these three factors interact. Therefore, if the environment is not very acceptable, the person will start to behave in an undesirable way, which emerges in the form of stress. This problem impacts people's behavior, emotions, cognitive performance, physical health, and psychological well-being. It poses a hazard to both the present and the future [87]. A multidisciplinary strategy incorporating the social, biological, and other sciences is needed to control this [87].

Therefore, the surrounding environment is one of the factors with significant effects on mental health and human stress, and humans react to environmental stimuli, which are called stressors. Environmental events threatening humans and causing stress are called environmental stressors. According to the research by Lazarus and Cohen [16], these factors are divided into three categories of cataclysmic events (sudden and unique events that affect a large number of people and are usually beyond the control of individuals or groups, such as natural disasters, war, etc.), stressful life events (life events or changes that affect fewer people or one person, such as a building collapse, etc.), and daily hassles (stable, repeated or chronic events, such as poverty, crowding, lack of hygiene, poor diet, etc.) [16]. The third category is considered the most important environmental stressors. Although it is not as dramatic as the other categories, it brings higher relative costs than other categories when occurring over time [16].

Many studies have addressed the impact of environmental stressors such as noise, temperature, light, and color on mental health, and some have related environmental stressors to social factors and raised issues such as crowding [88]. Burton [5] identified the following factors as environmental stressors.

- Exposure to chemicals (formaldehyde, carbon monoxide, SO_2, NO_2, toxic chemicals at work, additives).
- Exposure to physical factors (noise, ionizing and non-ionizing radiation, particles and smoke, climatic and geophysical hazards, secular architecture and urban design, housing conditions: temperature, ventilation, access to green spaces).
- Exposure to biological factors (microbes, viruses, bacteria, diet).
- Technological risks (car accidents, accidents at home, public transportation).
- Social, economic, and behavioral stressors (lack of exercise, obesity, excessive use of drugs, alcoholism, drug addiction, venereal disease, smoking, mental illness, suicide, lack of security, theft, crime, rape, domestic violence, unemployment, divorce, death of a close relative, lack of social support networks) [5].

2.9 Urbanization and Stress

As was previously noted, the global urban population is growing quickly, and by 2050, 64% of the world's population is predicted to live in cities. Numerous research in recent years have linked urbanisation to a risk for people's mental health, including stress and depression [84]. The environment, especially the built environment of the city, has a great impact on humans, and factors such as pollution, noise, crowding, extreme temperature, and so on are more in cities compared to villages. In metropolitan environments, environmental stresses like traffic may contribute to stress, which frequently manifests as medical ailment, mental disease, and decreased social contact [87]. If urban dwellers lack adequate living space, security, and stable economic situations, they will experience stress [30]. Urban life is generally regarded as stressful due to cities' pollution, unhygienic surroundings, monotony, exhaustion, and confusion. This is especially true for marginalised groups living in low-income, hazardous neighbourhoods with subpar living conditions and isolation [89]. The stress of city life causes some stress-related mental disorders in urban environments [90] and its impact is greater among low-income urbanites, especially the youth and teenagers [91]. But due to the importance of this issue, the impact of urban structure on stress and mental health disorders is not well known and few studies have addressed it [21]. Especially in developing countries where urbanization is growing at a very high speed, there is a need to pay more attention to the relationship between urban stress and mental health of citizens [92].

2.10 Urban Stress

The advantages of urban life have always attracted people to cities. On all continents, cities are economic, scientific, cultural, and political centers and are considered essential engines for social integration. However, the risk of stress-related mental illness is higher for urbanites than for rural dwellers [8]. Genetic risk factors can interact with education and social changes in the city to create and exacerbate mental diseases, such as stress and anxiety [93]. Urban and urbanising cultures are increasingly seen as facing the global mental health issue known as "urban stress" [94]. The precise nature of this phrase is still unclear despite its frequent use in scientific journals and the media. A greater grasp of this concept's nature appears to be a crucial component for advancement in this study field because it has not been thoroughly defined or investigated [95]. Below are a few definitions of urban stress:

- Urban life causes undesirable events such as pollution, high population, extreme temperature, crowding, noise, destroyed landscape, excessive accumulation of solid waste, waste of time in commuting, etc. and the city is a place where the most common stressful experiences happen. If these conditions are beyond a person's tolerance, it is said that the person experiences urban stress. Urban stress, as the relationship between the urban environment and its impact on the human condition, emphasizes the deterioration of the quality of the urban environment due to the increase in the urban population density, which leads to the deterioration of people's mental health [87].
- Urban residents and users are exposed to pollution, overcrowding, extreme temperatures, degraded landscapes, high levels of noise, etc. When this exposure exceeds the individual's tolerance, he may feel stressed [29].
- Urban stress is a general term related to the relationship between the urban context and its impact on the human condition, which is mostly related to the deterioration of the quality of the urban environment due to the increase in urban population density as a result of urbanization. This situation leads to the deterioration of people's mental health through urban life [84].
- Urban stress is the cumulative stress caused by the experience of living in unfavorable conditions of the urban environment because this environment is more stressful than the rural environment [27].
- Urban stress is a multifaceted concept because it may be caused by the combination of numerous stimuli, from visual, and auditory stimuli, unpredictable traffic, movement of population, or pollution, to more complex phenomena such as complex social interactions [72].
- Urban stress is a reaction to some threats perceived by urban factors [74].

According to the definitions presented above, the following definition of urban stress seems to be a comprehensive one:

Urban stress is the cumulative stress caused by the experience of living in unfavorable conditions of the urban environment and a general term related to the relationship between the urban environment and its impact on human mental health and a reaction to some threats perceived by undesirable urban events such as pollution, high population, extreme temperature, crowding, noise, destroyed landscape, excessive accumulation of solid waste, waste of time in commuting, etc., and if these conditions are beyond the urbanite's tolerance, he will experience urban stress.

2.11 The Relationship Between City, Health, Mental Health, and Stress

Considering the impact of urban life on mental health, a detailed understanding of the relationship between mental health and the city is required for urban planning and urban design, and to improve people's health and quality of life in urban environments, and a better understanding of this relationship helps to develop coping strategies and form future cities in a better way. To this end, after reviewing the theoretical background, this section attempts to describe the relationship between the city, health, mental health, and stress. As shown in Fig. 2.3, the relationship

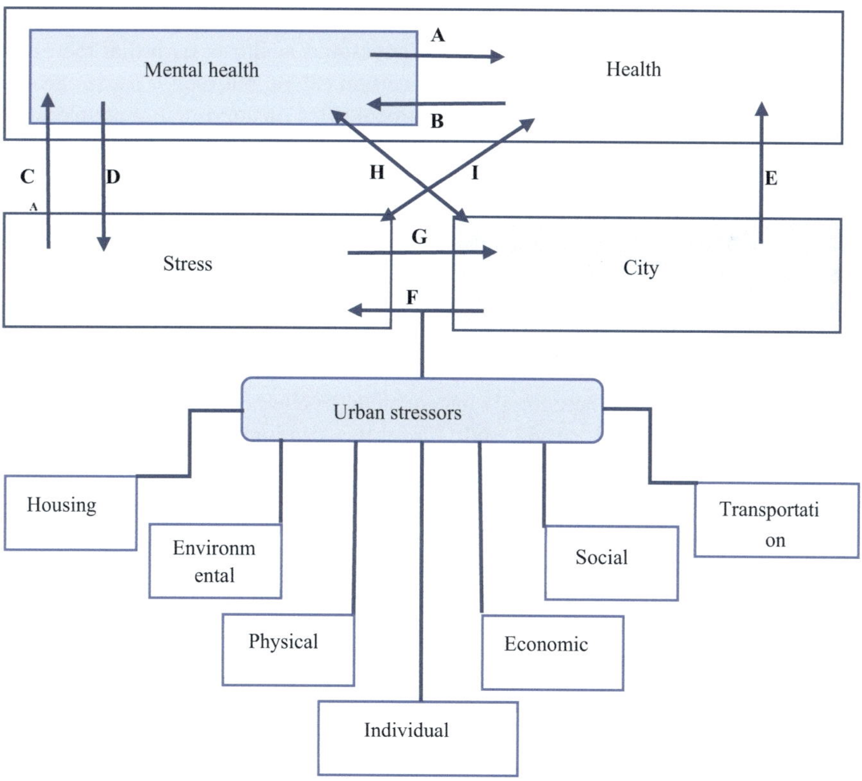

Fig. 2.3 Explaining the relationship between city, health, mental health, and stress

between these factors is not a complicated issue. Mental health is an important part of overall health and well-being and is very important for a healthy and happy life [96]. Since deteriorated health and physical diseases reduce the quality of mental health (B) and mental diseases also affect physical health (A), there is a mutual relationship between them [20].

Cities can have adverse and favorable consequences on health (E) and cause diseases such as diabetes, asthma, high blood pressure, etc. [15]. Also, they directly influence mental health (H) and reduce mental health [6]. In fact, exposure to a stressful environment such as the city significantly affects both physical and mental health [97]. Urbanites are exposed to higher levels of stressors and exposure to more stress may account for the prevalence of stress-related mental illness among urbanites [90]. Therefore, the city environment-induced stress (F) can deteriorate mental health [98]. Exposure to higher stress and the resulting injuries is the most important factor in increasing the risk of mental disorders [30]. New evidence shows that the stress of modern city life can be a ground for the emergence of psychosis and mental disorders [99]. Stress is a known risk factor for psychological injuries (C) [100].

Stress also influences health by causing cardiovascular and digestive diseases and reducing the immune system (I) [101]. Increasing the speed of aging and increasing the risk of aging-related diseases are other effects of stress on health [102]. Of course, the relationship between stress and health is such that the existence of stress helps to improve health to a certain extent, but then it causes health to diminish [5] and this relationship is reciprocal [5]. Considering that people with cognitive disorders, which are a type of mental illnesses, are more vulnerable to stress (D), mental health also has a significant impact on stress [86]. The effect of stress on the city (G) is unknown. In fact, since the stress of citizens affects their ability to work, it seems to be effective on the city and its economic resources in this way.

According to Fig. 2.3, the city both directly influences mental health and causes stress through social, economic, physical, environmental, housing, transportation, and individual stressors, and this stress reduces mental health. Of course, because physical and mental health are highly interrelated, the city also affects mental health by degrading general or physical health. The city is also impacted by mental health, both directly and indirectly through stress and public health. Therefore, the effects of urbanisation on mental health as well as the effects of mental health on the city might be mediated by urban stress and physical health. To make the most of urban life, it will be extremely helpful to have a greater understanding of this link, the role of mediators, and efforts to lessen the detrimental effects of cities on mental health.

2.12 Conclusion

This chapter describes the relevant terms and concepts to the book subject. The main findings of the present chapter include the introduction of the terms such as health, mental health, stress, and their relationship with the concepts of city and urbanization. Moreover, the most important finding of this chapter is the analysis of the relationship between these concepts through content analysis and Fig. 2.3. In fact, the city both influences mental health and causes stress through social, economic, physical, environmental, housing, transportation, and individual stressors, and this stress reduces mental health. Of course, the city also influences mental health through the reduction of general or physical health, because the areas of health and mental health are largely interdependent. Mental health also affects the city both directly and through stress and public health. As a result, urban stress and physical health can mediate the effects of urbanization on mental health and the effects of mental health on the city. A better understanding of this relationship and the effect of mediators and trying to reduce the negative effects of cities on mental health will greatly help to best take advantage of urban life.

References

1. Freudenberg N. Health promotion in the city: a review of current practice and future prospects in the United States. Annu Rev Public Health. 2000;21(1):473–503. https://doi.org/10.1146/annurev.publhealth.21.1.473.
2. Huber M, Knottnerus JA, Green L, Horst H, Jadad AR, Kromhout D, et al. How should we define health? BMJ. 2011;343(2):d4163. https://doi.org/10.1136/bmj.d4163.
3. French D. Residential segregation and health in Northern Ireland. Health Place. 2009;15(3):888–96. https://doi.org/10.1016/j.healthplace.2009.02.012.
4. Sellström E, Bremberg S. The significance of neighbourhood context to child and adolescent health and well-being: a systematic review of multilevel studies. Scand J Public Health. 2006;34(5):544–54. https://doi.org/10.1080/14034940600551251.
5. Burton I. Factors in urban stress. J Sociol Soc Welf. 1990;17(1):Article 5.
6. Evans BE, van der Ende J, Greaves-Lord K, Huizink AC, Beijers R, de Weerth C. Urbanicity, hypothalamic-pituitary-adrenal axis functioning, and behavioral and emotional problems in children: a path analysis. BMC Psychol. 2020;8:12. https://doi.org/10.1186/s40359-019-0364-2.
7. Nnebue ChC, Adinma ED, Queencallista N. Urbanization and health. Orient J Med. 2014;26.
8. Adli M, Schondorf J. Macht uns die Stadt krank. Wirkung von Stadtstress auf Emotionen, Verhalten und psychische Gesundheit; Does the city make us ill? The effect of urban stress on emotions, behavior, and mental health. Bundesgesundheitsbl. 2020;63:979–86. https://doi.org/10.1007/s00103-020-03185-w.
9. Kirkbride JB, Keyes KM, Susser E. City living and psychotic disorders—implications of global heterogeneity for theory development. JAMA Psychiatry. 2018;75:1211–2. https://doi.org/10.1001/jamapsychiatry.2018.2640.
10. Gruebner O, Rapp MA, Adli M, Kluge U, Galea S, Heinz A. Cities and mental health. Dtsch Arztebl Int. 2017;114:121–7. https://doi.org/10.3238/arztebl.2017.0121.
11. Okkels N, Kristiansen CB, Munk-Jørgensen P, Sartorius N. Urban mental health. Curr Opin Psychiatry. 2018;31:258–64. https://doi.org/10.1097/YCO.0000000000000413.
12. Semenza JC. The intersection of urban planning, art, and public health: the Sunnyside Piazza. Am J Public Health. 2003;93(9):1439–41. https://doi.org/10.2105/ajph.93.9.1439.
13. Ompad DC, Galea S, Vlahov D. Urban health systems: overview. In: Quah SR, editor. International encyclopedia of public health. 2nd ed. Academic. p. 311–7.
14. Douglas I. Ecosystems and human well-being. In: Reference module in earth systems and environmental sciences, encyclopedia of the anthropocene. Elsevier; 2015. p. 185–97. https://doi.org/10.1016/B978-0-12-409548-9.09206-X.

15. Sheila C, Oldroyd JC, Andre R. Urbanisation, urbanicity, and health: a systematic review of the reliability and validity of urbanicity scales. BMC Public Health. 2013;13:513.
16. Stephens C. Global issues: urban health in developing countries. In: Quah SR, Cockerham WC, editors. International encyclopedia of public health, vol. 3. 2nd ed. Elsevier.
17. Galea S, Freudenberg N, Vlahov D. Cities and population health. Soc Sci Med. 2005;60(5):1017–33.
18. Quah SR. Disability, illness and health risks: public health and epidemiology approaches. In: Reference module in biomedical sciences. Elsevier; 2018. https://doi.org/10.1016/B978-0-12-801238-3.66190-1.
19. Desai NG, Tiwari SC, Nambi S, Shah B, Singh RA, Kumar D, et al. Urban mental health services in India: how complete or incomplete? Indian J Psychiatry. 2004;46(3):195–212.
20. Lloyd S, Kelly R, Kimberly G, Joshua R. Challenges of urban mental health disaster planning. J Aggress Maltreat Trauma. 2005;10(3):695–706. https://doi.org/10.1300/J146v10n03_03.
21. Larcombe E, Logan P, Horwitz A. High-rise apartments and urban mental health—historical and contemporary views. Challenges. 2019;10(2):34. https://doi.org/10.3390/challe10020034.
22. Helbich M. Toward dynamic urban environmental exposure assessments in mental health research. Environ Res. 2018;161:129–35. https://doi.org/10.1016/j.envres.2017.11.006.
23. Joshua CF, Freeman C, Bazargan-Hejazi S. Environmental interventions for physical and mental health: challenges and opportunities for Greater Los Angeles. Int J Environ Res Public Health. 2019;16(12):2180. https://doi.org/10.3390/ijerph16122180.
24. Xie S. Quality matters: housing and the mental health of rural migrants in urban China. Hous Stud. 2019;2019:1–23. https://doi.org/10.1080/02673037.2019.1577956.
25. Scully C. Scully's medical problems in dentistry. Ment Health. 2014;2014:294–322. https://doi.org/10.1016/b978-0-7020-5401-3.00010-2.
26. Knight BG, Lee L. Mental health. In: Encyclopedia of gerontology. Elsevier; 2007. p. 159–66. https://doi.org/10.1016/B0-12-370870-2/00124-4.
27. Miller KM, Phillips MH. Correlates of urban stress and mental health: the impact of social context on resilience. J Soc Distress Homeless. 2005;14(1–2):46–64. https://doi.org/10.1179/105307805807066301.
28. Evans BE, Huizink AC, Greaves-Lord K, Tulen JHM, Roelofs K, van der Ende J, et al. Urbanicity, biological stress system functioning and mental health in adolescents. PLoS One. 2020;15(3):e0228659. https://doi.org/10.1371/journal.pone.0228659.
29. Kyriakou K, Resch B. Spatial analysis of moments of stress derived from wearable sensor data. Adv Cartogr GIScience Int Cartogr Assoc. 2019;2:9. https://doi.org/10.5194/ica-adv-2-9-2019.
30. Adli M. Urban stress and mental health. Cities, health and well-being, Hong Kong; 2011.
31. Krabbendam L, van Os J. Schizophrenia and urbanicity: a major environmental influence—conditional on genetic risk. Schizophr Bull. 2005;31(4):795–9. https://doi.org/10.1093/schbul/sbi060.
32. Corcoran R, Mansfield R, Giokas T, Hawkins A, Bamford L, Marshall G. Places change minds: exploring the psychology of urbanicity using a brief contemplation method. SAGE Open. 2017;7(2):215824401770700. https://doi.org/10.1177/2158244017707004.
33. Miles R, Coutts C, Mohamadi A. Neighborhood urban form, social environment, and depression. J Urban Health. 2012;89(1):1–18. https://doi.org/10.1007/s11524-011-9621-2.
34. Wang JL. Rural–urban differences in the prevalence of major depression and associated impairment. Soc Psychiatry Psychiatr Epidemiol. 2004;39(1):19–25. https://doi.org/10.1007/s00127-004-0698-8.
35. Rohrer JE, Borders TF, Blanton J. Rural residence is not a risk factor for frequent mental distress: a behavioral risk factor surveillance survey. BMC Public Health. 2005;5(1):46. https://doi.org/10.1186/1471-2458-5-46.
36. Caracci G. Urban mental health: an international survey. Int J Ment Health. 2006;35(1):39–45. https://doi.org/10.2753/imh0020-7411350103.

37. Lewis G, David A, Andréassson S, Allebeck P. Schizophrenia and city life. Lancet. 1992;340(8812):137–40. https://doi.org/10.1016/0140-6736(92)93213-7.
38. Lewis G, Booth M. Are cities bad for your mental health? Psychol Med. 1994;24(4):913–5. https://doi.org/10.1017/S0033291700029007.
39. Marcelis M, Navarro-Mateu F, Murray R, Selten J-P, Van Os J. Urbanization and psychosis: a study of 1942–1978 birth cohorts in The Netherlands. Psychol Med. 1998;28(4):871–9. https://doi.org/10.1017/s0033291798006898.
40. Paykel ES, Abbott R, Jenkins R, Brugha TS, Meltzer H. Urban–rural mental health differences in Great Britain: findings from the National Morbidity Survey. Psychol Med. 2000;30(2):269–80. https://doi.org/10.1017/s003329179900183x.
41. Schelin EM, Munk-Jørensen P, Olesen AV, Gerlach J. Regional differences in schizophrenia incidence in Denmark. Acta Psychiatr Scand. 2000;101(4):293–9. https://doi.org/10.1034/j.1600-0447.2000.101004293.x.
42. Ayuso-Mateos J, Vázquez-Barquero J, Dowrick C, Lehtinen V, Dalgard O, Casey P, et al. Depressive disorders in Europe: prevalence figures from the ODIN study. Br J Psychiatry. 2001;179(4):308–16. https://doi.org/10.1192/bjp.179.4.308.
43. Pedersen CB. Evidence of a dose-response relationship between urbanicity during upbringing and schizophrenia risk. Arch Gen Psychiatry. 2001;58(11):1039–46. https://doi.org/10.1001/archpsyc.58.11.1039.
44. Allardyce J, Boydell J, Van Os J, Morrison G, Castle D, Murray RM, McCreadie RG. Comparison of the incidence of schizophrenia in rural Dumfries and Galloway and urban Camberwell. Br J Psychiatry. 2001;179:335–9. https://doi.org/10.1192/bjp.179.4.335.
45. Harrison G, Fouskakis D, Rasmussen F, Tynelius P, Sipos A, Gunnell D. Association between psychotic disorder and urban place of birth is not mediated by obstetric complications or childhood socio-economic position: a cohort study. Psychol Med. 2003;33(4):723–31. https://doi.org/10.1017/s0033291703007591.
46. van Os J, Pedersen CB, Mortensen PB. Confirmation of synergy between urbanicity and familial liability in the causation of psychosis. Am J Psychiatry. 2004;161(12):2312–4. https://doi.org/10.1176/appi.ajp.161.12.2312.
47. Sundquist K, Frank G, Sundquist J. Urbanisation and incidence of psychosis and depression: follow-up study of 4.4 million women and men in Sweden. Br J Psychiatry. 2004;184(4):293–8. https://doi.org/10.1192/bjp.184.4.293.
48. Kovess-Masféty V, Alonso J, de Graaf R, Demyttenaere K. A European approach to rural—urban differences in mental health: The ESEMeD 2000 Comparative Study. Can J Psychiatr. 2005;50(14):926–36. https://doi.org/10.1177/070674370505001407.
49. Weich S, Twigg L, Lewis G. Rural/non-rural differences in rates of common mental disorders in Britain: prospective multilevel cohort study. Br J Psychiatry. 2006;188(1):51–7. https://doi.org/10.1192/bjp.bp.105.008714.
50. Pedersen CB, Mortensen PB. Are the cause(s) responsible for urban-rural differences in schizophrenia risk rooted in families or in individuals? Am J Epidemiol. 2006;163:971–8. https://doi.org/10.1093/aje/kwj169.
51. Peen J, Dekker J, Schoevers RA, Have M, de Graaf Ron B, Aartjan T. Is the prevalence of psychiatric disorders associated with urbanization? Soc Psychiatry Psychiatr Epidemiol. 2007;42(12):984–9.
52. Dekker J, Peen J, Koelen J, Smit F, Schoevers R. Psychiatric disorders and urbanization in Germany. BMC Public Health. 2018;8:17. https://doi.org/10.1186/1471-2458-8-17.
53. Heinz A, Deserno L, Reininghaus U. Urbanicity, social adversity and psychosis. World Psychiatry. 2013;12(3):187–97. https://doi.org/10.1002/wps.20056.
54. Haddad L, Schafer A, Streit F, Lederbogen F, Grimm O, Wust S, et al. Brain structure correlates of urban upbringing, an environmental risk factor for schizophrenia. Schizophr Bull. 2015;41(1):115–22. https://doi.org/10.1093/schbul/sbu072.
55. Vassos E, Agerbo E, Mors O, Pedersen CB. Urban-rural differences in incidence rates of psychiatric disorders in Denmark. Br J Psychiatry. 2016;208(5):435–40. https://doi.org/10.1192/bjp.bp.114.161091.

56. Knöll M, Neuheuser K, Cleff T, Rudolph-Cleff A. A tool to predict perceived urban stress in open public spaces. Environ Plan B Urban Anal City Sci. 2017;45:797–813. https://doi.org/10.1177/0265813516686971.
57. Toulopoulou T, Picchioni M, Mortensen PB, Petersen L. IQ, the urban environment, and their impact on future schizophrenia risk in men. Schizophr Bull. 2017;43(5):1056–63. https://doi.org/10.1093/schbul/sbw147.
58. Manning N. Sociology, biology and mechanisms in urban mental health. Soc Theory Health. 2018;17:1–22. https://doi.org/10.1057/s41285-018-00085-7.
59. Lee CK, Kwak YS, Yamamoto J, Rhee H, Kim YS, Han JH, et al. Psychiatric epidemiology in Korea. J Nerv Ment Dis. 1990;178(4):247–52.
60. Waqar H. Depression, anxiety, and stress among urban and rural police officers. J Police Crim Psychol. 2019;35:443–7. https://doi.org/10.1007/s11896-019-09358-x.
61. Coid J, Zhang Y, Li T. Urbanicity and psychosis in a Chinese undergraduate population: preliminary findings. Schizophr Bull. 2020;46(Supplement_1):S185–6. https://doi.org/10.1093/schbul/sbaa030.444.
62. Webb SD, Collette J. Rural-urban differences in the use of stress-alleviative drugs. Am J Sociol. 1977;83(3):700–7. https://doi.org/10.1086/226600.
63. McGrath J, Saha S, Welham J, El Saadi O, MacCauley C, Chant D. A systematic review of the incidence of schizophrenia: the distribution of rates and the influence of sex, urbanicity, migrant status and methodology. BMC Med. 2014;2:13. https://doi.org/10.1186/1741-7015-2-13.
64. DeVylder JE, Kelleher I, Lalane M, Oh H, Link BG, Koyanagi A. Association of urbanicity with psychosis in low- and middle-income countries. JAMA Psychiatry. 2018;75:678–86. https://doi.org/10.1001/jamapsychiatry.2018.0577.
65. Peen J, Schoevers RA, Beekman AT, Dekker J. The current status of urban-rural differences in psychiatric disorders. Acta Psychiatr Scand. 2010;121(2):84–93.
66. Colodro-Conde L, Couvy-Duchesne B, Whitfield JB, Streit F, Gordon S, Kemper K, et al. Association between population density and genetic risk for schizophrenia. JAMA Psychiatry. 2018;75(9):901–10. https://doi.org/10.1001/jamapsychiatry.2018.1581.
67. Vojnovic I, Pearson A, Asiki G, Allen A, DeVerteuil G. Handbook of global urban health. 1st ed. Routledge; 2019. https://doi.org/10.4324/9781315465456.
68. Wing J. Community and schizophrenia. By H. W. Dunham Detroit: Wayne State University Press. 1965. Pp. 312. Price $12.50. Br J Psychiatry. 1966;112(489):862. https://doi.org/10.1192/bjp.112.489.862.
69. Sampson L, Ettman CK, Galea S. Urbanization, urbanicity, and depression. Curr Opin Psychiatry. 2020;33(3):233–44. https://doi.org/10.1097/YCO.0000000000000588.
70. Li J, Rose N. Urban social exclusion and mental health of China's rural-urban migrants – a review and call for research. Health Place. 2017;48:20–30. https://doi.org/10.1016/j.healthplace.2017.08.009.
71. D'Acci LS. Urbanicity mental costs valuation: a review and urban-societal planning consideration. Mind Soc. 2020;9:223–35. https://doi.org/10.1007/s11299-020-00235-3.
72. Lilith AE, Baumann PS, Söderström O, Codeluppi Z, Söderström D, Conus P. Urbanicity: the need for new avenues to explore the link between urban living and psychosis. Early Interv Psychiatry. 2019;14:398–409. https://doi.org/10.1111/eip.12861.
73. Caracci G. General concepts of the relationship between urban areas and mental health. Curr Opin Psychiatry. 2008;21(4):385–90. https://doi.org/10.1097/yco.0b013e328303e198.
74. Ventriglio A, Torales J, Castaldelli-Maia JM, De Berardis D, Bhugra D. Urbanization and emerging mental health issues. CNS Spectr. 2020;2020:1–8. https://doi.org/10.1017/S1092852920001236.
75. Vaetisi S. Anti-urban ideologies and practices in the evolution of the American City. Anti-urbanism in America. Transylvanian Rev. 2013;3:82–95.
76. Srole L. Urbanization and mental health: some reformulations: anti-city biases of the past century are critically examined in the light of recent research evidence. Am Sci. 1972;60(5):576–83.

77. Fink G. Stress: definition and history. In: Squire L, editor. Encyclopedia of neuroscience. Elsevier; 2010. p. 549–55. https://doi.org/10.1016/B978-008045046-9.00076-0.
78. Jackson M. Stress in postwar Britain, 1945–1980. Pickering and Chatto; 2015.
79. McCay L, Bremer I, Endale T, Jannati M, Yi J. Urban design and mental health. In: Okkels N, Kristiansen CB, Munk-Jørgensen P, editors. Mental health and illness in the city. Springer; 2017. p. 421–44. https://doi.org/10.1007/978-981-10-2327-9_12.
80. Lazarus RS, Folkman S. Stress, appraisal and coping. New York: Springer; 1984.
81. Evans GW, Cohen S. Environmental stress. In: Overview of the stress paradigm. Elsevier; 1987. p. 571–602.
82. Benoit AC, Cotnam J, Raboud J, Greene S, Beaver K, Zoccole A, et al. Experiences of chronic stress and mental health concerns among urban Indigenous women. Arch Womens Ment Health. 2016;19(5):809–23. https://doi.org/10.1007/s00737-016-0622-8.
83. Baum AS, Jerome EB, Carlene S. Stress and the environment. Soc Issues. 1981;37(1):4–35. https://doi.org/10.1111/j.1540-4560.1981.tb01056.x.
84. Elsamahy EM, Abd El-Fattah R. Designing non-stressed psychological public spaces. BAU J Health Wellbeing. 2018;2018:121–32.
85. Quinn K, Kaufman JS, Siddiqi A, Yeatts KB. Stress and the city: housing stressors are associated with respiratory health among low socioeconomic status Chicago children. PLoS One. 2010;87(4):688–702. https://doi.org/10.1007/s11524-010-9465-1.
86. Baumann PS, Söderström O, Abrahamyan Empson L, Söderström D, Codeluppi Z, Golay P, et al. Urban remediation: a new recovery-oriented strategy to manage urban stress after first-episode psychosis. Soc Psychiatry Psychiatr Epidemiol. 2019;55:273–83. https://doi.org/10.1007/s00127-019-01795-7.
87. Rishi P, Khuntia G. Urban environmental stress and behavioral adaptation in Bhopal City of India. Urban Stud Res. 2012;2012:1–9. https://doi.org/10.1155/2012/635061.
88. Meloni A, Fornara F, Carrus G. Predicting pro-environmental behaviors in the urban context: the direct or moderated effect of urban stress, city identity, and worldviews. Cities. 2019;88:83–90. https://doi.org/10.1016/j.cities.2019.01.001.
89. Li J, Liu Z. Housing stress and mental health of migrant populations in urban China. Cities. 2018;81:172–9. https://doi.org/10.1016/j.cities.2018.04.006.
90. Adli M, Berger M, Brakemeier E-L, Engel L, Fingerhut J, Hehl R, et al. Neurourbanistik – ein methodischer Schulterschluss zwischen Stadtplanung und Neurowissenschaften. Die Psychiatrie. 2016;13:70–8.
91. Reynolds LK, O'Koon JH, Papademetriou E, Szczygiel S, Grant KE. Stress and somatic complaints in low-income urban adolescents. J Youth Adolesc. 2001;30(4):499–514. https://doi.org/10.1023/a:1010401417828.
92. Suchday S, Kapur S, Ewart CK, Friedberg JP. Urban stress and health in developing countries: development and validation of a neighborhood stress index for India. Behav Med. 2006;32(3):77–86. https://doi.org/10.3200/bmed.32.3.77-86.
93. Pykett J, Osborne T, Resch B. From urban stress to neurourbanism: how should we research city well-being? Ann Am Assoc Geogr. 2020;2020:1–16. https://doi.org/10.1080/24694452.2020.1736982.
94. Pykett J, Chrisinger B, Kyriakou K, Osborne T, Resch B, Stathi A, et al. Developing a citizen social science approach to understand urban stress and promote wellbeing in urban communities. Palgrave Commun. 2020;6:85. https://doi.org/10.1057/s41599-020-0460-1.
95. Abrahamyan Empson L, Baumann PS, Söderström O, Codeluppi Z, Söderström D, Conus P. Urbanicity: the need for new avenues to explore the link between urban living and psychosis. Early Interv Psychiatry. 2020;14(4):398–409. https://doi.org/10.1111/eip.12861.
96. McPherson KE, Kerr S, McGee E, Morgan A, Cheater FM, McLean J, et al. The association between social capital and mental health and behavioural problems in children and adolescents: an integrative systematic review. BMC Psychol. 2014;2:7. https://doi.org/10.1186/2050-7283-2-7.
97. Lederbogen F, Haddad L, Meyer-Lindenberg A. Urban social stress – risk factor for mental disorders. The case of schizophrenia. Environ Pollut. 2013;183:2–6. https://doi.org/10.1016/j.envpol.2013.05.046.

98. Wandersman A, Nation M. Urban neighborhoods and mental health. Psychological contributions to understanding toxicity, resilience, and interventions. Am Psychol. 1998;53(6):647–56.
99. Kennedy DP, Adolphs R. Social neuroscience: stress and the city. Nature. 2011;474(7352):452–3. https://doi.org/10.1038/474452a.
100. Streit F, Haddad L, Paul T, Frank J, Schäfer A, Nikitopoulos J, et al. A functional variant in the neuropeptide S receptor 1 gene moderates the influence of urban upbringing on stress processing in the amygdala. Stress. 2014;17(4):352–61. https://doi.org/10.3109/10253890.2014.921903.
101. McEwen BS, Stellar E. Stress and the individual mechanisms leading to disease. Arch Intern Med. 1993;153:2093–101.
102. Zannas AS, Arloth J, Carrillo-Roa T, Iurato S, Röh S, Ressler KJ, et al. Lifetime stress accelerates epigenetic aging in an urban, African American cohort: relevance of glucocorticoid signaling. Genome Biol. 2015;16:266. https://doi.org/10.1186/s13059-015-0828-5.

Chapter 3
Description of Urban Stressors

Abstract Since the city causes urban stress through urban stressors and influences the mental health of citizens, this chapter defines stressors and urban stressors. Then, the urban stressors are identified and analyzed through content analysis of previous studies.

Since urbanites face high levels of stressors and the resulting stress can reduce their mental health, it is very important to examine urban stressors as potential links between the aspects of the built environment and mental health. However, there has not been adequate research on urban stressors so far, and more studies have mentioned some of the stressors. Since it is very important to identify all the effective features of the urban context on mental health and stress and provide some solutions to reduce it in the development of stress-relief urban planning and design, this section aims to identify urban stressors by collecting data from documentary and library studies and analyzing them using categorical content analysis. In fact, using an interpretative approach (in several steps), the collected qualitative data was analyzed and then, these qualitative data were converted into quantitative ones to analyze them more easily by taking into account the repetition of each stressor.

Step 1. In this step, relevant research on mental health and urban stress was searched and reviewed. Then, irrelevant research was removed, and 42 research published from 1977 to 2021 were included.

Step 2. In this step, after considering urban stressors as subcategories, they, based on the similarities between them, are classified into land-use and activity, physical form (planning features, design features), transportation, environmental (climate, environmental pollution, environmental visibility, safety), social, economic, cultural, housing, and individual characteristics categories.

Step 3. After identifying the categories and subcategories in the previous step, the repetition percentage of the category is determined taking into account the frequency of each subcategory. Next, the findings are analyzed.

Keywords Environmental stress · Urban stress · Urban stressors · Content analysis

S. Jalilisadrabad et al., *Stress Relief Urban Planning*,
https://doi.org/10.1007/978-981-99-4202-2_3

3.1 Introduction

Since the city causes urban stress through urban stressors and influences the mental health of citizens, this chapter defines stressors and urban stressors. Then, the urban stressors are identified and analyzed through content analysis of previous studies.

3.2 Stressors

Stressors are considered to be stressful and pathogenic ground stimuli influencing a person, making him vulnerable to mental illnesses [1]. These factors have always been studied by psychologists, sociologists, and epidemiologists, etc. throughout history, and various types have been considered for them [2]. Lazarus and Cohen [3] considered three general categories of stressors, but as mentioned, they emphasized environmental stress and it did not include all factors [2]. Stressors can be divided into two types: external and internal stressors.

3.2.1 External Stressors

External stressors are environmental factors influencing humans and are also called environmental stressors [4]. Table 3.1 introduces these factors:

Table 3.1 External stressors [4]

External stressors	Natural stressors	All living or non-living things that occur naturally on earth, such as climate as high or low temperatures, rain, wind, and humidity, natural resources such as green areas, and natural disasters such as fires, floods, and earthquakes.	
	Human-made stressors	Physical stressors	They are tangible factors in the built environment, including the urban context, architectural building, and public urban spaces with all their physical elements
		Non-physical stressors	They are intangible factors, including civilization, society, and economic factors
		Social stressors	These factors are more related to human interaction and communication with other people, for example, issues such as peer group pressure, social isolation, life-changing events, family, and work, in addition to interaction with the surrounding environment such as overcrowding, noise, the traumatic effects of accidents, pollution, traffic jam, etc.

3.2.2 *Internal Stressors*

Internal stressors come from within the human body, including the following two main categories:

(a) Feelings: it refers to anything that can be experienced through human senses, such as touch, smell, sight, hearing, and taste. Feelings are often influenced by personal experience, beliefs, and memories such as hunger, hot, cold, disturbance, etc.
(b) Emotions: they are arising from the human body's reaction to external stimuli and have become a part of human genes during evolution. These emotions are the main stimuli that lead to stress. Humans require sensory experiences to understand the surrounding world, and they are formed using the five main human senses. These senses play an important role in transferring external stressors to the brain to take an action.

3.3 Urban Stressors

Living in a city, especially a big metropolis, is inexorably linked to increased stress levels. Early in the twentieth century, activity and density in expanding cities, as well as anonymity, were identified as elements affecting the human mind. However, there has not yet been adequate research on urban stressors and their remedies [5]. Urban stressors can be identified using three different methods: structural models, which emphasise macro-level indicators like poverty, unemployment, or crime for a large population; neighbourhood disorder models, which concentrate on neighbourhood-level indicators like social conflict, physical deterioration, and general decay; and environmental stress models, which look at ambient phenomena like noise, heat, or pollution. Of course, some studies have applied a combination of these models [6].

Since urbanites face high levels of stressors and the resulting stress can reduce their mental health, it is very important to examine urban stressors as potential links between the aspects of the built environment and mental health. However, there has not been adequate research on urban stressors so far, and more studies have mentioned some of the stressors. Since it is very important to identify all the effective features of the urban context on mental health and stress and provide some solutions to reduce it in the development of stress-relief urban planning and design, this section aims to identify urban stressors by collecting data from documentary and library studies and analyzing them using categorical content analysis. Using an interpretative approach, the collected qualitative data was analyzed and then, these qualitative data were converted into quantitative ones to analyze them more easily by taking into account the repetition of each stressor.

Step 1. In this step, relevant research on mental health and urban stress was searched and reviewed in Table 3.2. Then, irrelevant research was removed, and 42 research published from 1977 to 2021 were included.

Table 3.2 Introduces the stressors mentioned in these studies

	Cappon [7]	Burton [8]	Stansfeld et al. [9]	Caracci and Enrique Mezzich [10]	Evans et al. [11]	Jaffee et al. [12]	Selten [13]	Miller and Phillips [1]	March et al. [14]	Yang and Matthews [15]	Peen et al. [16]	Quinn et al. [17]	Adli [18]	Lin et al. [19]	Rishi and Khuntia [20]	Seth et al. [21]
Expert	1977	1990	2000	2001	2003	2005	2005	2005	2008	2010	2010	2010	2011	2011	2012	2012
Year															*	
Time pressure and waste of time																
Unhealthy lifestyle																
Improper diet	*	*	*								*		*		*	
Air pollution	*	*											*		*	
Water pollution		*											*		*	
Visual pollution										*					*	
Garbage accumulation and proximity to landfill sites																
Light pollution										*					*	
Traffic density																
Vehicle accidents																
High daily travel time	*			*				*								*
Facing violence	*		*			*		*		*	*					
Facing crime	*		*	*		*		*								
Job insecurity and unemployment																
Lack of economic support					*	*	*	*	*	*						

Lack of social capital					*	*	*	*	*	*						
Lack of social support					*							*			*	
Poor social interactions							*									
Social failure																
Low social cohesion																
Social stigma				*				*				*				*
Social deprivation				*					*			*				*
Economic deprivation									*							
Psychocultural deprivation	*						*	*								*
Social discrimination								*	*							
Social segregation	*		*					*	*		*					
Social isolation													*			
Social distinction	*							*								
Gentrification																
Lack of social diversity								*						*		
Injustice in the city					*					*		*				
Insecurity in the urban environment																
Long distances							*									
Migration							*		*							
Being of an ethnic or group minority	*			*		*		*		*						*

(continued)

Table 3.2 (continued)

	Cappon [7]	Burton [8]	Stansfeld et al. [9]	Caracci and Enrique Mezzich [10]	Evans et al. [11]	Jaffee et al. [12]	Selten [13]	Miller and Phillips [1]	March et al. [14]	Yang and Matthews [15]	Peen et al. [16]	Quinn et al. [17]	Adli [18]	Lin et al. [19]	Rishi and Khuntia [20]	Seth et al. [21]
Poverty	*	*	*						*	*	*	*	*		*	
Population density (too high or too low)	*	*	*							*	*		*		*	
Noise pollution															*	
Destroyed urban environment				*				*		*						*
Low socioeconomic status	*															
Very tall buildings																
Narrow roads with no escape route																
Endless cementation of space																
The presence of open space in non-walkable places																
Dilapidated and worn-out buildings																

Poor lighting of streets and urban environments																
Low quality of roads																
The presence of wide streets																
Lack of vegetation on the street																
Stressful squares																
The presence of big urban spaces																
The presence of spaces with no view																
Lack of sky view																
Large blocks																
Simple walls without details																
Lack of transparent facades																
The proximity of the housing to the high-traffic street																
Lack of pedestrian zone																
Lack of proper walking facilities																

(continued)

Table 3.2 (continued)

	Cappon [7]	Burton [8]	Stansfeld et al. [9]	Caracci and Enrique Mezzich [10]	Evans et al. [11]	Jaffee et al. [12]	Selten [13]	Miller and Phillips [1]	March et al. [14]	Yang and Matthews [15]	Peen et al. [16]	Quinn et al. [17]	Adli [18]	Lin et al. [19]	Rishi and Khuntia [20]	Seth et al. [21]
Lack of suitable furniture in streets and open spaces																
Inadequate public transportation																
Inappropriate access to resources and services																
Repetitive patterns in the built environment																
Infectious agents	*															
Lack of contact with nature												*				
The high number of residents per unit																
High building density																
Lack of facilities in society																
The identitylessness of the city																

Low sense of belonging																
Suppression of emotions in the city																
Lack of entertainment facilities													*			
Circadian rhythm disorders																
Language barriers of immigrant citizens		*	*		*			*				*				
The low quality of the residential unit					*					*						*
Residential instability																
Lack of home ownership																
The absence of a yard in the houses																
The small area of the residential unit					*											
Living on the upper floors					*											
The identitylessness of housing				*				*								
Homelessness			*					*								

(continued)

Table 3.2 (continued)

	Cappon [7]	Burton [8]	Stansfeld et al. [9]	Caracci and Enrique Mezzich [10]	Evans et al. [11]	Jaffee et al. [12]	Selten [13]	Miller and Phillips [1]	March et al. [14]	Yang and Matthews [15]	Peen et al. [16]	Quinn et al. [17]	Adli [18]	Lin et al. [19]	Rishi and Khuntia [20]	Seth et al. [21]
Perceiving the lack of control and prediction of the environment																
Lack of privacy												*				
Low security																
Lack of green space and poor access to it																
Inadequate quality of green space										*						*
Poor educational opportunities						*										*
Inadequate mental health services																*
Residential segregation																
Powerlessness in the city																
Perceiving a lower degree of respect for the whole community																
Chaos																

Suburbanization												*			*	
Urban heat islands and the high temperatures of the city			*					*		*						
Low income																
Being anonymous in the city																
Dealing with strangers																
High rent, land, and housing prices											*					
High mortality rate																
Drug exposure												*				
Difficult movement in the city																
Stressful urban design																
Modern architectural style								*								
Sensory overload (excessive sensory stimulation)									*							
Low participation of the residents in the city																

(continued)

Table 3.2 (continued)

	Cappon [7]	Burton [8]	Stansfeld et al. [9]	Caracci and Enrique Mezzich [10]	Evans et al. [11]	Jaffee et al. [12]	Selten [13]	Miller and Phillips [1]	March et al. [14]	Yang and Matthews [15]	Peen et al. [16]	Quinn et al. [17]	Adli [18]	Lin et al. [19]	Rishi and Khuntia [20]	Seth et al. [21]
Non-mixed land use																
The low literacy of people																
The abundance of child- and female-headed households					*											
Far from collective gathering places					*											
Ignoring suitable facilities for the disabled																
Lack of proper view of the city (up to 10 m)																
High global integration																
High citywide integration																
Low local integration																
Low axial connectivity																

Lack of spaces to enhance physical activity																
Lack of vitality in the urban environment																
High roundness ratio in urban space																
High openness ratio of an environment																
Dormitory-style environment																
The presence of a high percentage of the elderly in an environment	*															
Vulnerability to natural hazards	*															
Vulnerability to epidemics										*						
Food insecurity																
Drug abuse					*											
Improper lighting of the urban environment																
The inelegance of the environment																

(continued)

Table 3.2 (continued)

	Miles et al. [22]	Beil and Hanes [23]	Lederbogen et al. [24]	Hill and Maimon [25]	Knöll et al. [26]	Mubi Brighenti and Pavoni [27]	Li and Rose [28]	Gruebner et al. [29]	Knöll et al. [30]	Li and Liu [31]	Evans et al. [32]	Manning [33]	Generaal et al. [34]	Lisa and Ash [35]	Vojnovic et al. [36]
Expert	*2012*	*2013*	2013	2013	2014	2017	2017	2017	2017	2018	2018	2018	2019	2019	2019
Year															
Time pressure and waste of time															
Unhealthy lifestyle			*												
Improper diet			*		*			*	*			*	*		
Air pollution								*				*			
Water pollution												*			
Visual pollution															
Garbage accumulation and proximity to landfill sites			*		*										
Light pollution	*		*		*			*	*				*		*
Traffic density								*							
Vehicle accidents															
High daily travel time	*		*					*							
Facing violence	*	*		*											
Facing crime	*		*	*	*						*	*			
Job insecurity and unemployment	*														

Lack of economic support			*					*							
Lack of social capital			*					*							
Lack of social support	*			*		*	*			*					
Poor social interactions											*	*		*	
Social failure			*										*		
Low social cohesion														*	
Social stigma			*	*			*							*	
Social deprivation	*		*	*			*							*	
Economic deprivation							*								
Psychocultural deprivation							*								
Social discrimination							*	*							
Social segregation							*				*	*		*	
Social isolation															
Social distinction															
Gentrification															
Lack of social diversity							*			*		*			
Injustice in the city					*					*			*		*

(continued)

Table 3.2 (continued)

	Miles et al. [22]	Beil and Hanes [23]	Lederbogen et al. [24]	Hill and Maimon [25]	Knöll et al. [26]	Mubi Brighenti and Pavoni [27]	Li and Rose [28]	Gruebner et al. [29]	Knöll et al. [30]	Li and Liu [31]	Evans et al. [32]	Manning [33]	Generaal et al. [34]	Lisa and Ash [35]	Vojnovic et al. [36]
Insecurity in the urban environment															
Long distances				*			*					*		*	
Migration				*							*	*	*		
Being of an ethnic or group minority	*			*								*			
Poverty			*		*				*	*	*	*			*
Population density (too high or too low)	*	*	*		*			*	*	*		*	*		*
Noise pollution															
Destroyed urban environment							*	*							
Low socioeconomic status								*							
Very tall buildings															
Narrow roads with no escape route															
Endless cementation of space															*

The presence of open space in non-walkable places										*					
Dilapidated and worn-out buildings										*					*
Poor lighting of streets and urban environments										*					
Low quality of roads															*
The presence of wide streets															*
Lack of vegetation on the street															*
Stressful squares									*						*
The presence of big urban spaces															*
The presence of spaces with no view															
Lack of sky view									*						
Large blocks									*						*
Simple walls without details															*
Lack of transparent facades									*						*

(continued)

Table 3.2 (continued)

	Miles et al. [22]	Beil and Hanes [23]	Lederbogen et al. [24]	Hill and Maimon [25]	Knöll et al. [26]	Mubi Brighenti and Pavoni [27]	Li and Rose [28]	Gruebner et al. [29]	Knöll et al. [30]	Li and Liu [31]	Evans et al. [32]	Manning [33]	Generaal et al. [34]	Lisa and Ash [35]	Vojnovic et al. [36]
The proximity of the housing to the high-traffic street									*						
Lack of pedestrian zone															*
Lack of proper walking facilities					*										*
Lack of suitable furniture in streets and open spaces															*
Inadequate public transportation				*			*			*					
Inappropriate access to resources and services															
Repetitive patterns in the built environment															
Infectious agents		*													
Lack of contact with nature		*													
The high number of residents per unit	*								*						*

High building density		*													
Lack of facilities in society						*	*			*					
The identitylessness of the city							*								
Low sense of belonging						*									
Suppression of emotions in the city						*									
Lack of entertainment facilities															
Circadian rhythm disorders														*	
Language barriers of immigrant citizens							*			*				*	
The low quality of the residential unit	*			*											
Residential instability															
Lack of home ownership									*						
The absence of a yard in the houses					*										

(continued)

Table 3.2 (continued)

	Miles et al. [22]	Beil and Hanes [23]	Lederbogen et al. [24]	Hill and Maimon [25]	Knöll et al. [26]	Mubi Brighenti and Pavoni [27]	Li and Rose [28]	Gruebner et al. [29]	Knöll et al. [30]	Li and Liu [31]	Evans et al. [32]	Manning [33]	Generaal et al. [34]	Lisa and Ash [35]	Vojnovic et al. [36]
The small area of the residential unit															
Living on the upper floors															
The identitylessness of housing															
Homelessness										*					
Perceiving the lack of control and prediction of the environment										*					
Lack of privacy	*									*					*
Low security	*		*		*				*				*		
Lack of green space and poor access to it															*
Inadequate quality of green space			*				*								
Poor educational opportunities			*				*								
Inadequate mental health services															

Residential segregation															
Powerlessness in the city							*								
Perceiving a lower degree of respect for the whole community											*				
Chaos															
Suburbanization									*						
Urban heat islands and the high temperatures of the city	*			*			*				*		*		
Low income											*				
Being anonymous in the city											*				
Dealing with strangers															
High rent, land, and housing prices															
High mortality rate															
Drug exposure															
Difficult movement in the city															
Stressful urban design															*

(continued)

Table 3.2 (continued)

	Miles et al. [22]	Beil and Hanes [23]	Lederbogen et al. [24]	Hill and Maimon [25]	Knöll et al. [26]	Mubi Brighenti and Pavoni [27]	Li and Rose [28]	Gruebner et al. [29]	Knöll et al. [30]	Li and Liu [31]	Evans et al. [32]	Manning [33]	Generaal et al. [34]	Lisa and Ash [35]	Vojnovic et al. [36]
Modern architectural style															
Sensory overload (excessive sensory stimulation)	*						*								
Low participation of the residents in the city	*														*
Non-mixed land use	*			*											
The low literacy of people	*														
The abundance of child- and female-headed households															
Far from collective gathering places															
Ignoring suitable facilities for the disabled									*						*
Lack of proper view of the city (up to 10 m)									*						*

High global integration									*						*
High citywide integration									*						*
Low local integration									*						
Low axial connectivity			*						*						
Lack of spaces to enhance physical activity					*										*
Lack of vitality in the urban environment									*						
High roundness ratio in urban space									*						
High openness ratio of an environment															
Dormitory-style environment	*														
The presence of a high percentage of the elderly in an environment															
Vulnerability to natural hazards															

(continued)

Table 3.2 (continued)

	Miles et al. [22]	Beil and Hanes [23]	Lederbogen et al. [24]	Hill and Maimon [25]	Knöll et al. [26]	Mubi Brighenti and Pavoni [27]	Li and Rose [28]	Gruebner et al. [29]	Knöll et al. [30]	Li and Liu [31]	Evans et al. [32]	Manning [33]	Generaal et al. [34]	Lisa and Ash [35]	Vojnovic et al. [36]
Vulnerability to epidemics															
Food insecurity															
Drug abuse															
Improper lighting of the urban environment															
The inelegance of the environment															

	Interdisciplinary Forum Neurourbanism [37]	Xie [38]	Abrahamyan Empson et al. [39]	Baumann et al. [40]	Meloni et al. [41]	Vargas et al. [42]	D'Acci [43]	Adli and Schondorf [5]	Pykett et al. [44]	Ventriglio [45]	Litman [46]
Expert	2019	2019	2019	2019	2019	2020	2020	2020	2020	2020	2021
Year										*	
Time pressure and waste of time										*	
Unhealthy lifestyle										*	
Improper diet			*	*	*				*	*	*
Air pollution			*	*	*					*	
Water pollution			*	*	*					*	
Visual pollution											
Garbage accumulation and proximity to landfill sites			*								*
Light pollution			*		*					*	*
Traffic density											
Vehicle accidents										*	
High daily travel time			*						*	*	
Facing violence						*				*	*
Facing crime		*								*	*
Job insecurity and unemployment											

(continued)

Table 3.2 (continued)

	Interdisciplinary Forum Neurourbanism [37]	Xie [38]	Abrahamyan Empson et al. [39]	Baumann et al. [40]	Meloni et al. [41]	Vargas et al. [42]	D'Acci [43]	Adli and Schondorf [5]	Pykett et al. [44]	Ventriglio [45]	Litman [46]
Lack of economic support			*	*						*	*
Lack of social capital			*	*						*	*
Lack of social support	*	*	*	*						*	*
Poor social interactions			*	*		*					
Social failure											
Low social cohesion		*								*	
Social stigma		*		*		*		*	*	*	
Social deprivation				*		*					*
Economic deprivation											
Psychocultural deprivation		*							*	*	
Social discrimination	*					*				*	
Social segregation	*							*	*	*	*
Social isolation										*	
Social distinction	*										
Gentrification	*										
Lack of social diversity		*				*				*	*
Injustice in the city										*	*
Insecurity in the urban environment										*	

Long distances		*	*	*						*	
Migration			*	*		*		*		*	
Being of an ethnic or group minority								*			*
Poverty	*			*	*	*	*	*	*	*	
Population density (too high or too low)			*	*	*			*	*	*	*
Noise pollution					*						
Destroyed urban environment											
Low socioeconomic status			*								
Very tall buildings			*								
Narrow roads with no escape route							*				
Endless cementation of space											
The presence of open space in non-walkable places											
Dilapidated and worn-out buildings									*		
Poor lighting of streets and urban environments											

(continued)

Table 3.2 (continued)

	Interdisciplinary Forum Neurourbanism [37]	Xie [38]	Abrahamyan Empson et al. [39]	Baumann et al. [40]	Meloni et al. [41]	Vargas et al. [42]	D'Acci [43]	Adli and Schondorf [5]	Pykett et al. [44]	Ventriglio [45]	Litman [46]
Low quality of roads											
The presence of wide streets											
Lack of vegetation on the street											
Stressful squares											
The presence of big urban spaces											
The presence of spaces with no view							*				
Lack of sky view											
Large blocks											
Simple walls without details											
Lack of transparent facades											
The proximity of the housing to the high-traffic street											
Lack of pedestrian zone											*
Lack of proper walking facilities											

Lack of suitable furniture in streets and open spaces											*
Inadequate public transportation								*			*
Inappropriate access to resources and services									*		
Repetitive patterns in the built environment			*								
Infectious agents										*	*
Lack of contact with nature											
The high number of residents per unit											
High building density											
Lack of facilities in society											
The identitylessness of the city						*					
Low sense of belonging											
Suppression of emotions in the city											

(continued)

Table 3.2 (continued)

	Interdisciplinary Forum Neurourbanism [37]	Xie [38]	Abrahamyan Empson et al. [39]	Baumann et al. [40]	Meloni et al. [41]	Vargas et al. [42]	D'Acci [43]	Adli and Schondorf [5]	Pykett et al. [44]	Ventriglio [45]	Litman [46]
Lack of entertainment facilities											
Circadian rhythm disorders		*									
Language barriers of immigrant citizens		*							*	*	
The low quality of the residential unit		*									
Residential instability		*									
Lack of home ownership											
The absence of a yard in the houses		*									
The small area of the residential unit		*									
Living on the upper floors											
The identitylessness of housing										*	*
Homelessness											

Perceiving the lack of control and prediction of the environment										*	*
Lack of privacy						*					
Low security				*			*			*	
Lack of green space and poor access to it											
Inadequate quality of green space						*					*
Poor educational opportunities										*	
Inadequate mental health services											
Residential segregation									*		
Powerlessness in the city											
Perceiving a lower degree of respect for the whole community									*		
Chaos										*	
Suburbanization								*			
Urban heat islands and the high temperatures of the city								*	*		

(continued)

Table 3.2 (continued)

	Interdisciplinary Forum Neurourbanism [37]	Xie [38]	Abrahamyan Empson et al. [39]	Baumann et al. [40]	Meloni et al. [41]	Vargas et al. [42]	D'Acci [43]	Adli and Schondorf [5]	Pykett et al. [44]	Ventriglio [45]	Litman [46]
Low income											
Being anonymous in the city											
Dealing with strangers								*			
High rent, land, and housing prices											
High mortality rate				*						*	
Drug exposure	*			*							
Difficult movement in the city				*							
Stressful urban design											
Modern architectural style				*							*
Sensory overload (excessive sensory stimulation)	*										
Low participation of the residents in the city											
Non-mixed land use											*
The low literacy of people											

The abundance of child- and female-headed households											
Far from collective gathering places											*
Ignoring suitable facilities for the disabled											
Lack of proper view of the city (up to 10 m)											
High global integration											
High citywide integration											
Low local integration											
Low axial connectivity										*	*
Lack of spaces to enhance physical activity							*				
Lack of vitality in the urban environment											
High roundness ratio in urban space											

(continued)

Table 3.2 (continued)

	Interdisciplinary Forum Neurourbanism [37]	Xie [38]	Abrahamyan Empson et al. [39]	Baumann et al. [40]	Meloni et al. [41]	Vargas et al. [42]	D'Acci [43]	Adli and Schondorf [5]	Pykett et al. [44]	Ventriglio [45]	Litman [46]
High openness ratio of an environment							*				
Dormitory-style environment											
The presence of a high percentage of the elderly in an environment											
Vulnerability to natural hazards											
Vulnerability to epidemics											
Food insecurity				*						*	
Drug abuse											
Improper lighting of the urban environment	*										
The inelegance of the environment	*										

Step 2. In this step, after considering urban stressors as subcategories, they, based on the similarities between them, are classified into land use and activity, physical form (planning features, design features), transportation, environmental (climate, environmental pollution, environmental visibility, safety), social, economic, cultural, housing, and individual characteristics categories.

Step 3. After identifying the categories and subcategories in the previous step, the repetition percentage of the category is determined taking into account the frequency of each subcategory. Next, the findings are analyzed. The final results are listed in Table 3.3.

As seen in Table 3.3, the experts in this field consider urban stress to be mostly caused by social stressors (36.67%) and environmental stressors (18.43%), followed by economic stressors (9.41%), stressors associated with the physical form (8.43%), transportation (7.06%), land-use and activity (6.67%), and housing (6.67%), cultural stressors (3.92%), and individual stressors (2.74%), respectively.

In the land-use and activity category, the lack of green space and poor access to it, and poor educational opportunities with higher repetition percentages were known as the most important stressors.

In the physical form category, the effective planning features of the environment on urban stress have been mostly proposed by the experts, and the stressors associated with the design features of the environment have been given less attention.

Table 3.3 Classification of urban stressors and the repetition percentage of each stressor

Category	Sub-category	Frequency	Repetition percentage	
Land-use and activity	Non-mixed land use	2	0.39	6.67
	Dormitory-style environment	1	0.20	
	Inappropriate access to resources and services	5	0.98	
	Lack of facilities in society	1	0.20	
	Lack of entertainment facilities	1	0.20	
	Inadequate mental health services	5	0.98	
	Lack of green space and poor access to it	8	1.57	
	Inadequate quality of green space	1	0.20	
	Lack of spaces to enhance physical activity	4	0.78	
	Lack of proper educational opportunities	6	1.18	

(continued)

Table 3.3 (continued)

Category		Sub-category	Frequency	Repetition percentage		
Physical form	**Planning features**	The presence of open space in non-walkable places	1	0.20	6.27	8.43
		Time pressure and waste of time	2	0.39		
		The presence of big urban spaces	2	0.39		
		Circadian rhythm disorders	1	0.20		
		Injustice in the city	9	1.76		
		Suburbanization	1	0.20		
		High roundness ratio[a] in the urban environment	1	0.20		
		High openness ratio[b] in an environment	1	0.20		
		The presence of very tall buildings	3	0.59		
		Poor lighting of streets and urban environments	3	0.59		
		Lack of suitable furniture in streets and open spaces	2	0.39		
		Ignoring suitable facilities for the disabled	2	0.39		
		The presence of very large blocks	1	0.20		
		High building density	3	0.59		
	Design features	The presence of dilapidated and worn-out buildings	1	0.20	2.16	
		Destroyed urban environment	2	0.39		
		The inelegance of the environment	1	0.20		
		Endless cementation of space	1	0.20		
		Lack of transparent facades	1	0.20		
		The presence of simple walls without details	2	0.39		
		Repetitive patterns in the built environment	1	0.20		
		Stressful urban design	1	0.20		
		Modern architectural style	1	0.20		

Table 3.3 (continued)

Category	Sub-category		Frequency	Repetition percentage		
Transportation	Narrow roads with no escape route		1	0.20		7.06
	Stressful squares		1	0.20		
	Traffic density		13	2.55		
	Vehicle accidents		1	0.20		
	High daily travel time		1	0.20		
	Long distances		1	0.20		
	Low quality of roads		1	0.20		
	The presence of wide streets		1	0.20		
	Lack of vegetation on the street		1	0.20		
	Inadequate public transportation		2	0.39		
	Difficult movement in the city		3	0.59		
	High global integration (r = n)[c]		2	0.39		
	High citywide integration (r = 3000 m)[d]		2	0.39		
	High axial connection[e]		1	0.20		
	Lack of walkable areas		1	0.20		
	Lack of proper walking facilities		2	0.39		
	Low local integration (r = 1200 m)[f]		2	0.39		
Environmental	**Climate**	Heat islands and high temperature	4	0.78	0.98	18.43
		Improper lighting of the urban environment	1	0.20		
	Environmental pollution	Infectious agents	1	0.20	14.71	
		Air pollution	18	3.53		
		Noise pollution	24	4.71		
		Light pollution	4	0.78		
		Visual pollution	8	1.57		
		Water pollution	10	1.96		
		Garbage accumulation and proximity to landfill sites	2	0.39		
		Lack of control and prediction of the environment	3	0.59		
		Sensory overload (excessive sensory stimulation)[g]	3	0.59		
		Chaos in the environment	2	0.39		
	Environmental vision	The presence of spaces with no view	1	0.20	1.37	
		Lack of sky view	1	0.20		
		Lack of proper view of the city (up to 10 m)	2	0.39		
		Lack of privacy	3	0.59		
	Security	Low security	5	0.98	1.37	
		Vulnerability to epidemics	1	0.20		
		Vulnerability to natural hazards	1	0.20		

(continued)

Table 3.3 (continued)

Category	Sub-category	Frequency	Repetition percentage	
Social	Lack of social capital[h]	12	2.35	36.67
	Lack of social support[i]	12	2.35	
	Poor social interactions[j]	14	2.75	
	Social failure[k]	7	1.37	
	Low social cohesion[l]	2	0.39	
	Social stigma[m]	3	0.59	
	Social deprivation[n]	14	2.75	
	Social discrimination[o]	8	1.57	
	Social segregation[p]	7	1.37	
	Social isolation[q]	14	2.75	
	Social Distinction[r]	2	0.39	
	Gentrification[s]	3	0.59	
	Migration	9	1.76	
	Lack of social diversity	1	0.20	
	Powerlessness in the city	1	0.20	
	Perceiving a lower degree of respect for the whole community	1	0.20	
	Dealing with strangers in the neighborhood	1	0.20	
	Population density (too high or too low)	24	4.71	
	The presence of a high percentage of the elderly in an environment	1	0.20	
	The abundance of a child- and female-headed households	1	0.20	
	Language barriers of immigrant citizens	2	0.39	
	Far from collective gathering places	1	0.20	
	Lack of vitality in the urban environment	3	0.59	
	Lack of security in the urban environment	9	1.76	
	The low literacy of people	3	0.59	
	High mortality rate	1	0.20	
	Suppression of emotions in the city	1	0.20	
	Drug exposure	2	0.39	
	Drug abuse	2	0.39	
	Low participation of the residents	4	0.78	
	Facing violence	10	1.96	
	Facing crime	12	2.35	
Economic	Lack of economic support	1	0.20	9.41
	Economic deprivation	12	2.35	
	Poverty	11	2.16	
	Job insecurity and unemployment	14	2.75	
	Low income	10	1.96	

Table 3.3 (continued)

Category	Sub-category	Frequency	Repetition percentage	
Cultural	Psychocultural deprivation	2	0.39	3.92
	Lack of cultural institutions and places	1	0.20	
	The identitylessness of the city	3	0.59	
	Low sense of belonging	2	0.39	
	Being of an ethnic or group minority	11	2.16	
	Being anonymous in the city	1	0.20	
Housing	The proximity of the housing to the high-traffic street	2	0.39	6.67
	The high number of residents per unit	2	0.39	
	The low quality of the residential unit	11	2.16	
	Residential instability	6	1.18	
	Lack of home ownership	1	0.20	
	The absence of a yard in the house	1	0.20	
	The small area of the residential unit	2	0.39	
	The identitylessness of housing	1	0.20	
	Homelessness	4	0.78	
	Residential segregation	1	0.20	
	High rent, land, and housing prices	1	0.20	
	Living on the upper floors	2	0.39	
Individual features	Unhealthy lifestyle	1	0.20	2.74
	Food insecurity	1	0.20	
	Low socioeconomic status	6	1.18	
	Lack of contact with nature	4	0.78	
	Improper diet	2	0.39	
		510	100	100

[a] It is obtained by dividing the isovist area by the square of the perimeter [47]
[b] It is defined as the balance between the closed and open edges of an isovist, which is related to interestingness and complexity [30]. It is obtained by dividing the square of the isovist perimeter by its area [47]. It refers to the relative visibility of the isovist area [30]
[c] High levels of accessibility at the global level or higher volumes of car traffic [30]
[d] The degree of integration of particular street segments in the urban grid has been considered a pervasive indicator for pedestrian movement patterns. It refers to high levels of access at the urban level or high urban traffic [30]
[e] It is defined the number of segments that are directly connected to a given street segment. High values in axial connectivity are co-linear with high densities of intersections [30]
[f] It refers to the low levels of accessibility at the local level [30]
[g] When secondary stimuli such as sound, light, etc. cannot be prevented and cause distraction, stimulation, and disturbance, a person is subjected to sensory overload [48]
[h] It is a part of the umbrella term intellectual capital and it refers to collective abilities resulting from social networks [49]. It includes all commitments, interactions, participation, relationships and interest that bind people of a society together [50]
[i] Supportive interactions among people are protective against health consequences of life stress [51]
[j] It refers to the relationship between two or more people that leads to a reaction between them [52]

(continued)

Table 3.3 (continued)

[k] It refers to the feeling of failure in the struggle and loss of social status or failure to achieve social resources [53]

[l] It is a kind of feeling of connection, desire, and tendency between people and it refers to the feeling of mutual responsibility between one or more people or several groups [54]

[m] It refers to the tarnishing of one's social identity due to which one is discredited and humiliated [55]

[n] Social deprivation includes different levels and aspects such as people's access to work, education, housing, skills, and private and public spaces. People who lack these things and do not have proper citizenship rights are called socially deprived [56]

[o] An act that intentionally violates social participation or human rights for a group of people [57]

[p] It refers to a set of social activities that are carried out by a social institution and cause a gap in society [58]

[q] It refers to the lack of a person's relationships with other people and groups in society so that he feels that he does not belong to that society [59]

[r] It means to be different and distinctive, or in other words, to have a distinguishing characteristic [60]

[s] It refers to the displacement of working-class residents of a neighborhood or urban fabric by the wealthier people [61]

Also, injustice in the city was known as the most frequent stressor associated with planning features and destroyed the urban environment, and simple walls without details were known as the most frequent stressor associated with the design features of the environment. It should be noted that all stressors associated with design features and most stressors associated with planning features have very low repetition percentages.

In the transportation category, traffic density with a repetition percentage of (2.55) was known as the most frequent stressor associated with transportation, and other factors had very low repetition percentages.

In the environmental category, the subcategory of environmental pollution (14.71%) was known as the most important stressor, followed by environmental visibility (1.37%), safety (1.37%), and climate (0.98%), respectively. Also, noise pollution and air pollution were known as the most frequent environmental stressors.

In the social category, population density (very high or very low) (4.71%) was known as the most frequent social stressor, followed by social isolation, social deprivation, and poor social interactions (2.75%). Also, job insecurity and unemployment in the economic category, low quality of the residential unit in the housing category, being an ethnic or group minority in the cultural category, and low socioeconomic status in the category of individual characteristics were recognized as the most frequent stressors. Comparing subcategories indicates that population density (very high or very low) and noise pollution (4.71%), are the most frequent subcategories. Therefore, they are the most important urban stressors, followed by air pollution (3.53%) and social isolation, social deprivation, poor social interactions, and job insecurity and unemployment (2.75%), respectively. Therefore, studies on urban stress have mostly addressed social and environmental stressors, and there is a need to identify and study other types of stressors.

3.4 Conclusion

As a result, previous studies in this field consider urban stress to be mostly induced by social stressors such as population density (too high or too low), social isolation, social deprivation, and poor social interactions, and environmental stressors such as noise pollution and air pollution. In fact, urban stress is mostly caused by population density and high noise pollution in urban environments, followed by job insecurity and unemployment in the economic field. Although the physical form of the urban environment is one of the other important factors affecting urban stress, few studies have mentioned the links between the city form and stress, and the studies in this field have emphasized planning factors such as injustice in the city and paid less attention to the design features of the city body. Next, high traffic density has been mentioned as the most frequent urban stressor in the field of transportation, followed by the lack of green space and poor access to it, poor educational opportunities in the dimension of land-use and activity, the low quality of residential units in the housing dimension, being an ethnic or group minority in the cultural dimension, and low socioeconomic status in the dimension of individual characteristics. In fact, what causes urban stress to be high in cities compared to villages are social and environmental factors. Of course, other factors are also very important and policy-makers, planners, designers, and architects should take a step to reduce the stressors abovementioned in urban environments after properly recognizing them.

References

1. Miller KM, Phillips MH. Correlates of urban stress and mental health: the impact of social context on resilience. J Soc Distress Homeless. 2005;14(1–2):46–64. https://doi.org/10.1179/105307805807066301.
2. Baum AS, Jerome EB, Carlene S. Stress and the environment. Soc Issues. 1981;37(1):4–35. https://doi.org/10.1111/j.1540-4560.1981.tb01056.x.
3. Lazarus RS, Cohen JB. Environmental stress. Hum Behav Environ. 1977;1977:89–127. https://doi.org/10.1007/978-1-4684-0808-9_3.
4. Elsamahy EM, Abd El-Fattah R. Designing non-stressed psychological public spaces. BAU J Health Well-Being. 2018;2018:121–32.
5. Adli M, Schondorf J. Macht uns die Stadt krank. Wirkung von Stadtstress auf Emotionen, Verhalten und psychische Gesundheit; Does the city make us ill? The effect of urban stress on emotions, behavior, and mental health. Bundesgesundheitsbl. 2020;63:979–86. https://doi.org/10.1007/s00103-020-03185-w.
6. Suchday S, Kapur S, Ewart CK, Friedberg JP. Urban stress and health in developing countries: development and validation of a neighborhood stress index for India. Behav Med. 2006;32(3):77–86. https://doi.org/10.3200/bmed.32.3.77-86.
7. Cappon D. Urban stress. CMA J. 1977;116:8.
8. Burton I. Factors in urban stress. J Sociol Soc Welf. 1990;17(1):Article 5.
9. Stansfeld S, Haines M, Brown B. Noise and health in the urban environment. Rev Environ Health. 2000:15(1–2). https://doi.org/10.1515/REVEH.2000.15.1-2.43.

10. Caracci G, Enrique MJ. Culture and urban mental health. Psychiatr Clin North Am. 2001;24(3):581–93. https://doi.org/10.1016/S0193-953X(05)70249-5.
11. Evans GW, Wells NM, Moch A. Housing and mental health: a review of the evidence and a methodological and conceptual critique. J Soc Issues. 2003;59(3):475–500. https://doi.org/10.1111/1540-4560.00074.
12. Jaffee KD, Liu GC, Canty-Mitchell J, Qi RA, Austin J, Swigonski N. Race, urban community stressors, and behavioral and emotional problems of children with special health care needs. Psychiatr Serv. 2005;56(1):63–9. https://doi.org/10.1176/appi.ps.56.1.63.
13. Selten JP. Social defeat: risk factor for schizophrenia? Br J Psychiatry. 2005;187(2):101–2. https://doi.org/10.1192/bjp.187.2.101.
14. March D, Hatch SL, Morgan C, Kirkbride JB, Bresnahan M, Fearon P, et al. Psychosis and place. Epidemiol Rev. 2008;30(1):84–100. https://doi.org/10.1093/epirev/mxn006.
15. Yang T, Matthews SA. The role of social and built environments in predicting self-rated stress: a multilevel analysis in Philadelphia. Health Place. 2010;16(5):803–10. https://doi.org/10.1016/j.healthplace.2010.04.005.
16. Peen J, Schoevers RA, Beekman AT, Dekker J. The current status of urban-rural differences in psychiatric disorders. Acta Psychiatr Scand. 2010;121(2):84–93.
17. Quinn K, Kaufman JS, Siddiqi A, Yeatts KB. Stress and the city: housing stressors are associated with respiratory health among low socioeconomic status Chicago children. PLoS One. 2010;87(4):688–702. https://doi.org/10.1007/s11524-010-9465-1.
18. Adli M. Urban stress and mental health. Cities, health and well-being, Hong Kong; 2011.
19. Lin D, Li X, Bo W, Yan H, Xiaoyi F, Xiong Q, Bonita S. Discrimination, perceived social inequity, and mental health among rural-to-urban migrants in China. Commun Ment Health. 2011;47(2):171–80. https://doi.org/10.1007/s10597-009-9278-4.
20. Rishi P, Khuntia G. Urban environmental stress and behavioral adaptation in Bhopal City of India. Urban Stud Res. 2012;2012:1–9. https://doi.org/10.1155/2012/635061.
21. Seth P, Murray CC, Braxton ND, DiClemente RJ. The concrete jungle: city stress and substance abuse among young adult African American Men. J Urban Health. 2012;90(2):307–13. https://doi.org/10.1007/s11524-012-9716-4.
22. Miles R, Coutts C, Mohamadi A. Neighborhood urban form, social environment, and depression. J Urban Health. 2012;89(1):1–18. https://doi.org/10.1007/s11524-011-9621-2.
23. Beil K, Hanes D. The influence of urban natural and built environments on physiological and psychological measures of stress. A pilot study. Int J Environ Res Public Health. 2013;10:1250–67. https://doi.org/10.3390/ijerph10041250.
24. Lederbogen F, Haddad L, Meyer-Lindenberg A. Urban social stress – risk factor for mental disorders. The case of schizophrenia. Environ Pollut. 2013;183:2–6. https://doi.org/10.1016/j.envpol.2013.05.046.
25. Hill TD, Maimon D. Neighborhood context and mental health. In: Aneshensel CS, Phelan JC, Bierman A, editors. Handbook of the sociology of mental health. Handbooks of sociology and social research; 2013. https://doi.org/10.1007/978-94-007-4276-5_23.
26. Knöll M, Neuheuser K, Vogt J, Rudolph-Cleff A. Einflussfaktoren der gebauten Umwelt auf wahrgenommene Aufenthaltsqualität bei der Nutzung städtischer Räume. Umweltpsychologie. 2014;18:84–102. https://www.researchgate.net/publication/270759025.
27. Mubi Brighenti A, Pavoni A. City of unpleasant feelings. Stress, comfort and animosity in urban life. Soc Cult Geogr. 2017;2017:1–20. https://doi.org/10.1080/14649365.2017.1355065.
28. Li J, Rose N. Urban social exclusion and mental health of China's rural-urban migrants – a review and call for research. Health Place. 2017;48:20–30. https://doi.org/10.1016/j.healthplace.2017.08.009.
29. Gruebner O, Rapp MA, Adli M, Kluge U, Galea S, Heinz A. Cities and mental health. Dtsch Arztebl Int. 2017; https://doi.org/10.3238/arztebl.2017.0121.

30. Knöll M, Neuheuser K, Cleff T, Rudolph-Cleff A. A tool to predict perceived urban stress in open public spaces. Environ Plan B Urban Anal City Sci. 2017; https://doi.org/10.1177/0265813516686971.
31. Li J, Liu Z. Housing stress and mental health of migrant populations in urban China. Cities. 2018; https://doi.org/10.1016/j.cities.2018.04.006.
32. Evans BE, Buil JM, Burk WJ, Cillessen AHN, van Lier PAC. Urbanicity is associated with behavioral and emotional problems in elementary school-aged children. J Child Fam Stud. 2018; https://doi.org/10.1007/s10826-018-1062z.
33. Manning N. Sociology, biology and mechanisms in urban mental health. Soc Theory Health. 2018;17:1–22. https://doi.org/10.1057/s41285-018-00085-7.
34. Generaal E, Hoogendijk EO, Stam M, Henke CE, Rutters F, Oosterman M, et al. Neighbourhood characteristics, prevalence, and severity of depression: pooled analysis of eight Dutch cohort studies. Br J Psychiatry. 2019;2019:1–8. https://doi.org/10.1192/bjp.2019.100.
35. Lisa R, Ash A. Mental health, subjectivity and the city: an ethnography of migrant stress in Shanghai. Int Health. 2019; https://doi.org/10.1093/inthealth/ihz029.
36. Vojnovic I, Pearson A, Asiki G, Allen A, DeVerteuil G. Handbook of global urban health. 1st ed. Routledge; 2019. https://doi.org/10.4324/9781315465456.
37. Interdisciplinary Forum Neurourbanism. Charta of Neurourbanism. 2018. https://neurourbanistik.de. Accessed 23 Sept 2021.
38. Xie S. Quality matters: housing and the mental health of rural migrants in urban China. Hous Stud. 2019;2019:1–23. https://doi.org/10.1080/02673037.2019.1577956.
39. Abrahamyan Empson L, Baumann PS, Söderström O, Codeluppi Z, Söderström D, Conus P. Urbanicity: the need for new avenues to explore the link between urban living and psychosis. Early Interv Psychiatry. 2019; https://doi.org/10.1111/eip.12861.
40. Baumann PS, Söderström O, Abrahamyan Empson L, Söderström D, Codeluppi Z, Golay P, et al. Urban remediation: a new recovery-oriented strategy to manage urban stress after first-episode psychosis. Soc Psychiatry Psychiatr Epidemiol. 2019; https://doi.org/10.1007/s00127-019-01795-7.
41. Meloni A, Fornara F, Carrus G. Predicting pro-environmental behaviors in the urban context: the direct or moderated effect of urban stress, city identity, and worldviews. Cities. 2019;88:83–90. https://doi.org/10.1016/j.cities.2019.01.001.
42. Vargas T, Conley RE, Mittal VA. Chronic stress, structural exposures and neurobiological mechanisms: a stimulation, discrepancy and deprivation model of psychosis. In: Clow A, Smyth N, editors. International review of neurobiology; 2020. p. 41–69. https://doi.org/10.1016/bs.irn.2019.11.004.
43. D'Acci LS. Urbanicity mental costs valuation: a review and urban-societal planning consideration. Mind Soc. 2020;9:223–35. https://doi.org/10.1007/s11299-020-00235-3.
44. Pykett J, Osborne T, Resch B. From urban stress to neurourbanism: how should we research city well-being? Ann Am Assoc Geogr. 2020;2020:1–16. https://doi.org/10.1080/24694452.2020.1736982.
45. Ventriglio A, Torales J, Castaldelli-Maia JM, De Berardis D, Bhugra D. Urbanization and emerging mental health issues. CNS Spectr. 2020;2020:1–8. https://doi.org/10.1017/S1092852920001236.
46. Litman TA. Urban sanity understanding urban mental health impacts and how to create saner. Happier Cities; 2021. https://vtpi.org/urban-sanity.pdf.
47. Franz G, Wiener JM. From space syntax to space semantics: a behaviorally and perceptually oriented methodology for the efficient description of the geometry and topology of environments. Environ Plann B Plann Des. 2008;35(4):574–92. https://doi.org/10.1068/b33050.
48. Scheydt S, Müller Staub M, Frauenfelder F, Nielsen GH, Behrens J, Needham I. Sensory overload: a concept analysis. Int J Ment Health Nurs. 2017;26(2):110–20. https://doi.org/10.1111/inm.12303.

49. Young J. Personal knowledge capital. In: Social capital and trust for a web environment; 2012. p. 81–90. https://doi.org/10.1016/b978-1-84334-700-2.50007-5.
50. Shirkhani M, Vaseiezadeh NS. Social capital and economic development: a comparative study of Iran and South Korea. Polit Q. 2011;41(2):213–32. Persian.
51. Schwarzer C. Encyclopedia of applied psychology. Soc Support. 2004;2004:435–41. https://doi.org/10.1016/b0-12-657410-3/00414-1.
52. Mansoor Mahani S. The impact of social interactions on architecture and urban public space. In: Annual Conference on Architecture, Urban Planning and Urban Management Research. Period 1, 2014. Persian.
53. Taylor PJ, Gooding P, Wood AM, Tarrier N. The role of defeat and entrapment in depression, anxiety, and suicide. Psychol Bull. 2011;137(3):391–420. https://doi.org/10.1037/a0022935.
54. Allen B. Culture of social sciences. Translated by Sarokhani B. Tehran: Kayhan Publications; 1996. Persian.
55. Ebadollahi H, Piri A, Movaghar Narbin M. Stigma and social identity: the case of individuals with visible physical disabilities in Rasht. Soc Probl Iran. 2012;2:195–222. Persian.
56. Thorns DC. The transformation of cities: urban theory and urban life. Springer; 2002. https://doi.org/10.1007/978-1-4039-9031-0.
57. Amiri M, Vedadhir A. Stigma and discrimination: two vital social oppressions influencing on disclosure of HIV status by patients with HIV/AIDS. Soc Probl Iran. 2018;8:1–23. Persian. https://doi.org/10.22059/ijsp.2018.65051.
58. Lahsayeezadeh AA, Khajeh Noori B. A critical study of the views of functionalists on social differentiation. J Soc Sci. 2004;1(3) https://doi.org/10.22067/jss.v0i0.3077. Persian.
59. Chalabi M, Amir Kafi M. Multilevel analysis of social isolation. Iran J Soc. 2004;5:3–31. Persian.
60. Bodat Y, Maroofi M. The impact of cultural and economic capitals on social distinction: with an emphasis on ownership of a luxury car. Refahj. 2017;17(65):137–70. Persian.
61. Hammel DJ. International encyclopedia of human geography. Gentrification. 2009;2009:360–7. https://doi.org/10.1016/b978-008044910-4.01051-8.

Chapter 4
Explaining Strategies to Reduce Urban Stress

Abstract Mental illnesses are caused by systemic problems, so, they require systemic solutions (Cerrato and Halamka, Ment Health 2019:115, 2019). The correction of these diseases requires interaction between factors such as environment, family, person, etc. (Evans et al., J Child Fam Stud 9, 2018). Considering the significant role of urban spaces in mental health, designers, architects, planners, policy-makers, and city managers should strive in this direction (Elsamahy and Abd El-Fattah, BAU J Health Well-Being 2018:132, 2018). This chapter, first, addresses how to deal with and reduce urban stress, and then, explains each of the solutions to reduce urban stress. Out of effective solutions to reduce urban stress, one can refer to holding mental health promotion workshops, improving access to mental health services, improving lighting in homes and urban spaces, improving the accessibility and quality of green spaces, developing and implementing a comprehensive mental health plan, Mental health-enhancing urban design, reducing time wastage and time pressure on citizens, promoting urban therapeutic gardening, controlling population density and building density, promoting urban resilience, promoting identity and sense of belonging to the city, revitalizing cultural and religious rituals, promoting social support and reducing social deprivation, leisure activities, promoting local integration, promoting people's control over the environment, applying the principles of smart growth and new urbanism, not using outdated styles such as modern style, reducing economic deprivation, reducing pollution in urban environments, promoting justice, encouraging proper diet and reducing malnutrition, promoting diversity in the urban environment, and implementing urban remediation strategies, as described below. To control urban stress, developing coping skills and implementing strategies to improve the environment, are of particular importance.

Keywords Environmental stress · Urban stress · Urban design · Urban remediation · Mental health

S. Jalilisadrabad et al., *Stress Relief Urban Planning*,
https://doi.org/10.1007/978-981-99-4202-2_4

4.1 Introduction

Mental illnesses are caused by systemic problems, so, they require systemic solutions [1]. The correction of these diseases requires interaction between factors such as environment, family, person, etc. [2]. Considering the significant role of urban spaces in mental health, designers, architects, planners, policymakers, and city managers should strive in this direction [3]. This chapter, first, addresses how to deal with and reduce urban stress, and then, explains each of the solutions to reduce urban stress.

4.2 Solutions to Reduce Urban Stress

The holding of mental health promotion workshops, enhancing access to mental health services, enhancing lighting in homes and urban areas, enhancing accessibility and the quality of green spaces, developing and implementing a comprehensive mental health plan, are just a few examples of practical ways to lessen urban stress. Designing cities in a way that promotes mental health, minimising time waste and time pressure on residents, encouraging therapeutic urban gardening, managing population and building density, fostering urban resilience, fostering sense of identity and belonging in the city, and reviving cultural and religious rituals, fostering community support and reducing social deprivation, leisure pursuits, local integration, fostering people's control over the environment, implementing smart growth and new urbanism principles, avoiding the use of outmoded fashions like modern style, reducing economic deprivation, reducing pollution in urban environments, fostering justice, encouraging a healthy diet and preventing malnutrition, fostering diversity in the urban environment, and implementing urban racial planning. To control urban stress, developing coping skills and implementing strategies to improve the environment, are of particular importance. Figure 4.1 shows the causes and consequences of stress in the urban environment (UES[1] model) and how to deal with it to achieve subjective well-being [4].

4.2.1 *Holding Mental Health Promotion Workshops*

Holding mental health promotion workshops can be considered a way to build capacity and develop innovative concepts to promote mental health and reduce urban stress. Also, these workshops promote the identity and sense of belonging to the city by fostering dialogue and expanding the social relations of people,

[1] Urban Environmental Stress and Health.

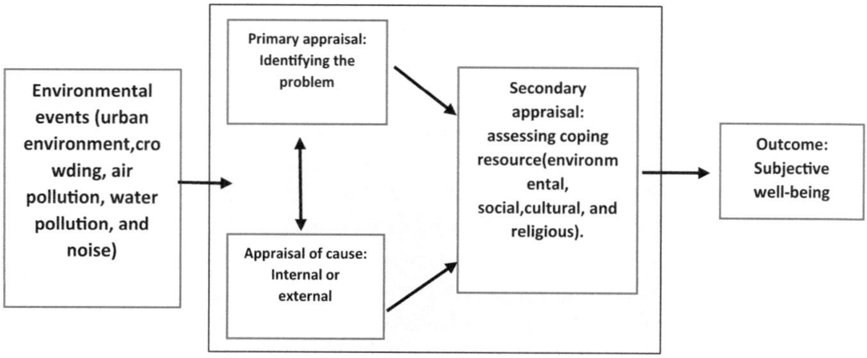

Fig. 4.1 An eclectic model of UES and coping with subjective well-being [4]

especially immigrants and ethnic minorities, ultimately promoting the participation of citizens [5].

4.2.2 Improving Access to Mental Health Services

The wide healthcare gap for mental disorders was raised in the 2000s and closing this gap was promoted as an urgent issue for health systems worldwide [6]. Studies have shown that in many urban environments, mental health services are not available or inadequate, or not optimally used due to the healthcare providers' misunderstanding of cultural differences, citizens' fear of the stigma associated with mental illness, and insufficient insurance coverage, etc. [7]. Governmental and non-governmental organizations play an important role in creating services and gutturalizing the optimal use of these services through political, religious, and academic institutions [7]. Also, since it is not possible for all people to receive face-to-face healthcare services and many people have no tendency to receive them, innovative approaches such as mobile health programs and online services seem useful [1].

4.2.3 Improving the Lighting of Houses and Urban Spaces

Cities have a higher rate of vitamin D insufficiency than rural places do, despite vitamin D being one of the key nutrients for mental wellness [8]. The variation in the prevalence of mental diseases between cities and rural areas may be caused in part by this problem. Light levels, especially exposure to daylight, have a variety of psychological consequences [9]. Therefore, enhancing the lighting in homes and urban areas can be a useful strategy for enhancing mental health and lowering urban stress.

4.2.4 Improving the Accessibility and Quality of Green Space

Urban green spaces are considered areas where many people daily contact with nature. Such contact has many physical and psychological advantages [10]. According to numerous studies, living in greener cities is associated with lower levels of psychological distress and improved mental well-being across communities. Green spaces may also be protective against stress. Additionally, due to lower levels of traffic-related air pollution, more exposure to green spaces is linked to better early childhood neurodevelopment [11]. Additionally, having access to green space reduces the negative and stressful effects of moving, and moving to greener metropolitan areas has been linked to consistent increases in mental health. As other benefits of green spaces, one can mention encouraging physical activity and promoting social relations [12]. In addition, green spaces reduce the effects of urban heat islands and heat stress and can moderate the stressful effects of tall buildings [13].

The difference between places with high and low socioeconomic social statuses will be narrowed by promoting environmental diversity (a natural environment made up of trees, plants, grasses, and species richness), especially in cities where there is an issue with land and resource shortages. Additionally, for high-rise apartments without balconies, measures such as creating "green streets," "living walls," "common rooftop gardens," "common green space around the apartment," and "encouraging the use of plants in the indoor environment" are advised [14]. Therefore, greening cities has environmental, economic, and psychological effects [15]. In addition to this, the physical, social, etc. effects are also considered the important effects of these spaces.

The relationship between green space and mental well-being has been explained by a number of theories, including the biophilic theory (based on the unconscious biological attitude of humans), the stress reduction theory (emphasizing the reduction of daily pressure-induced physiological and psychological stress with green spaces), and the attention restoration theory (emphasizing the need to pay more attention to and focus on green spaces) [11]. Also, many studies in different parts of the world have emphasized the positive effect of green spaces on stress. For example, one can refer to the studies by Beil and Hanes [16], Hazer et al. [17], Herrera et al. [18], Van den Berg et al. [19], Yang et al. [20], Miles et al. [21], Weeland et al. [22], Rishi and Khuntia [4], Abrahamyan Empson et al. [23], Maas et al. [24], Neale et al. [25], etc.

4.2.5 Developing and Implementing a Comprehensive Mental Health Plan

Cities need a database as a starting point. This detailed database is responsible for understanding available resources, structural strengths and weaknesses, available services, most common injuries, and specific needs of the population. This database forms the necessary foundation and bases for developing and implementing a comprehensive mental health plan for each city. Such a plan should take into account the cultural, economic, and social differences of residents and include strategies to reduce urban stress [7]. Also, this plan should specify the challenges and opportunities of future studies and require city managers to support relevant research. Gruebner et al. identified the most important challenges and opportunities, which are presented in Fig. 4.2.

To promote urban mental health, it is required to carried out longitudinal studies to analyze the relationship between the duration of exposure to the city and mental health.

Lack of information about the coping resources of the neighborhood (such as green spaces, etc.) and their effects on mental health and urban stress.

How to distribute effective urban resources in reducing stress and promoting mental health in a more fair, stable, and balanced way.

How to help explain the differences between groups and prevent issues such as discrimination and social or ethnic segregation, and assess their effects.

Enhancing knowledge in the field of interventions reducing urban stress in developing countries.

Interdisciplinary research between architecture, urban planning, epidemiology, geography, neuroscience, and sociology is essencial to understanding how the urban environment affects the mental health of populations. Only such an approach makes it possible to identify the populations who lack urban advantage and who are at risk.

Fig. 4.2 The most important challenges and opportunities for future research on the comprehensive mental health plan of cities [13]

4.2.6 Mental Health-Promoing Urban Design

The design of the built environment through physical stimuli (form, color, texture, sound, and light) has significant effects on emotions, cognition, behavior, and ultimately psychological well-being [26]. Urban design influences our perception by affecting the aesthetic aspects of a city, and this perception depends on four factors: sufficient complexity of the landscape, high coherence, easy legibility, and a certain degree of mystery that arouses curiosity and the need for exploration [26]. Urban design is a factor that promotes mental health because it may provide some places for recreational activities, relaxation, promoting social support, promoting security, and facilitating access to health care [11]. Also, using strategies such as using physical barriers in buildings, bridges, railways, and subways makes it possible to control suicide, which is one of the results of mental illnesses [11]. Urban design may also affect crime and violence rates [17]. Urban furniture also greatly influences mental health, so its proper design and location are very important. Among other factors affecting mental health in urban design, one can refer to unbeautiful and heterogeneous facades, so the beauty, attractiveness, cleanness, and compatibility of facades with native and cultural factors can be effective in improving mental health. Also, urban design plays an effective role in reducing and controlling several stressors mentioned in Table 3.2 such as very tall buildings, narrow streets without escape routes, endless cementation of space, lack of vegetation on the street, simple walls without details, repetitive patterns in the built environment, etc.

4.2.7 Reducing Time Wastage and Time Pressure on Citizens

Cities are potentially great places to live and achieve our goals and progress in our lives, individually and collectively. But urbanites are facing more stress caused by time pressure and time wastage, which can be reduced by urban planning and socio-economic lifestyles such as remote work plus flexible working hours, nationally reducing in weekly working hours, reducing waiting times at public transport stations, reducing the distance between work and living environment and services, etc. [15]. Using urban games is a good strategy to help travelers and people waiting in the traffic line to reduce their stress caused by time wastage. Of course, the type of games suggested must have strict criteria so that they don't endanger people's health [27].

4.2.8 Promoting Urban Therapeutic Gardening

Spending time and gardening in urban green environments designed for these purposes can help reduce stress, depression, and anxiety and improve the quality of life [28]. The concept of horticultural therapy refers to an intervention based on the activities and experiences of growing and harvesting plants in a natural environment to promote interaction with the natural environment and improve health [28]. Also, gardening activities play a significant role in improving mood and self-confidence [28]. The United States Department of Agriculture (USDA) launched an urban gardening programme in six locations in 1977, which the locals collectively oversaw. Additionally, the Housing and Community Development Commission of Columbia approved this programme for all of the province's public housing in 1978. This program emphasized the gardening of flowers and edible vegetables and resulted in enhanced self-confidence, revived neighborhoods, increased sociability, reduced vandalism, improved abandoned lands, revived public buildings, reduced urban stress, improved sense of belonging, and improved identity of citizens with poor socioeconomic status [29].

4.2.9 Control of Population Density and Building Density

Different techniques can be used to measure density. According to Söderström et al. [30], it is primarily either looked at as a demographic phenomenon or as a phenomenon connected to the built environment. Urban density, as opposed to urban sprawl, provides better access to services (including parks, playgrounds, health, and social care), which has been linked to improved mental health [13]. However, excessive population density and crowding of the urban environment are important stressors, and a balanced density should be considered in urban planning [31]. High building density is also one of the important causes of urban stress due to the lack of space, mass building, and the great number of floors. That is why proper control of building density is one of the effective solutions in this field [32].

4.2.10 Improving Urban Resilience

Researchers have found that providing information about how to deal with a stressor before people encounter it reduces the threat caused [33], making society resilient, improving a society's ability to resist past and future hardships, and strengthening belief in this ability, are considered a very important measure and a difficult part of mental health planning during a disaster [34]. Urban resilience refers to the ability of a city or an urban system to withstand stresses and shocks. The criteria for promoting resilience in an urban place are as follows: minimizing exposure to social stress, promoting social cohesion and a sense of belonging, enabling acquisition processes, and increasing the experience of environmental mastery [31].

Distinctive characteristics of a city must be considered when preparing for a mental health disaster. In addition, special and vulnerable populations with special needs (for example, refugees, the homeless, children, the elderly, and people with mental retardation, developmental disabilities, chemical dependencies, or mental illnesses) should also be considered in urban resilience [34].

4.2.11 Promoting Identity and Sense of Belonging to the City

Local identity at the city level can be a variable moderating urban stress. It can be assessed by items such as, I am proud to be from this city, I don't feel a part of my city's traditions, My city is not special compared to others, I feel a part of this city, and this city fascinates me [35]. Urban identity is felt when urban inhabitants have a strong desire to answer the question "Who am I?" by the group of citizens [36].

The sense of belonging and acquaintance increase residents' commitment to a neighborhood, and in the process of revitalizing a community, there must be a deep commitment to the neighborhood in such a way as to create a desire for changes in the residents. Instead of staying and improving the environment, most people look for ways to physically escape from it, and promoting a sense of belonging is the best solution to prevent this physical escape [37]. The physical escape of people or in other words migration itself is a risk factor for mental illness [38].

4.2.12 Revitalizing Cultural and Religious Rituals

Understanding these belief systems and incorporating these approaches into the modern system may be an effective way to promote mental health in cities. Communicating with supernatural forces and enacting rituals are needed to balance biological needs, spiritual harmony, and personal and cultural attachments. Additionally, addressing cultural demands and comprehending the ways in which cultural dynamics are portrayed to understand adaptation to urban living may substantially improve our capacity to accurately identify and treat mental illnesses in cities. In order to assess, treat, and lessen urban stress in mental patients living in metropolitan regions, contextual cultural elements are crucial [39].

4.2.13 Promoting Social Support and Reducing Social Deprivation

Numerous studies and pieces of evidence focus on the connections between the social environment and mental health since social coping is the most popular and personal form of coping across all social classes [4, 21]. Indeed, social connections and social support have a favourable impact on mental health [40], and social cohesion and social control operate as mediators between the negative impacts of urbanisation on mental health and urban stress [41]. The ability of a community to deal with the cumulative exclusion factors associated with living in urban neighbourhoods is decreased when there are positive social interactions amongst members of the community [37]. Enhancing social capital has a significant impact on mental health as well [42]. The most crucial methods for enhancing a community's social capital include the creation of social support networks (such as peer support), civic engagement in local institutions (such as volunteering), initiatives to raise literacy rates and educational standards, social cohesion, and social control [36]. The neighbourhood's physical environment has a significant influence in fostering social capital [43]. Also, installing artistic features, making places for social interactions [44], and residential segregation in the form of shared communities [45] will expand social networks among residents and stimulate their mental well-being. Promoting purposeful social services to reduce social stress caused by poverty, homelessness, immigration, etc. should be prioritized [11]. Because the consequences of social and economic deprivation are very wide. The healthcare costs associated with social and economic deprivation in the UK have been estimated at over £5.5 billion per year, which is only part of the economic consequences of this issue [46].

4.2.14 Leisure Activities

Leisure activities such as having fun, attending social and religious gatherings, participating in art workshops, doing physical sports, etc., are effective ways to overcome stress and achieve mental well-being [4]. In fact, laughing and laughter therapy during these activities can be significantly effective in improving mental health.

4.2.15 Promoting Local Integration

Walkable neighborhoods and areas with high local integration are less perceived as stressful [47]. People who live in pro-social, walkable neighborhoods report lower levels of psychological distress, lower crime rates, lower obesity rates, and lower rates of chronic disease. Creating lively and sociable environments that are clean, and pleasant, and promote walking and social interaction among people, sustainable public transportation, environments encouraging exercise, access to drinkable springs, providing places to sit, and extensive connectivity of local streets are effective measures promoting local integration [48].

4.2.16 Improving People's Control Over the Environment

People who maintain that they have control over their surroundings, regardless of whether they have it or not, experience less environmental stress. Designers, planners, and urban politicians should strive to create a predictable and controllable urban environment [49]. People feel better when they control their surroundings and feel helpless when they do not have the opportunity to control environmental features such as noise or pollution [9].

4.2.17 Applying the Principles of Smart Growth and New Urbanism

Smart growth and new urbanism movements have created neighbourhood environments that value more traditional elements including higher density, continuous street networks, mixed-use development, and accessibility to parks and public transportation. These features increase the opportunity for social interaction with neighbors and reduce dependence on personal cars by promoting livability and sustainability and supporting walking. Advocates of these approaches emphasize their benefits for mental health. Social interactions among neighborhood residents while walking, the presence of parks and green spaces, and physical activity resulting from walking lead to the improved mental health of citizens [21]. Also, urban sprawl and the development of the city to the periphery are associated with the increase in the rate of secondary diseases, immobility, increase in pollution, and loss of social capital, which are considered in these approaches [50]. Aiming to improve people's quality of life and build healthy communities through the design of successful urban public spaces so people can access areas without any limits, changing from a machine-oriented city to a city for people is one of the most crucial issues [3].

4.2.18 Not Using Outdated Styles Such as Modern Style

Due to stressors and negative life events like crowded and polluted environments, poverty and reliance on the cash economy, high levels of violence, a decline in social support, soulless environments, etc., modern urbanisation may have detrimental effects on mental health. Therefore, while designing a city, ample natural areas should be included as buffers against pollution (noise, dust, etc.) and as a lovely area for enjoyment and raising the standard of the environment [4]. In reality, the effects of modern architecture's repeating patterns on the sense of sight and cognitive processing may be detrimental to mental health [51].

4.2.19 Reducing Economic Deprivation

Evidence suggests that the number of poor people living in urban areas is increasing [52]. The problems dealt with by the urban poor have many psychological and social effects that lead to urban stress [53]. Immigrant groups increase the risk of poverty depending on their pre-immigration background and social stress [54]. In general, the economic deprivation of a neighborhood is strongly associated with residents' depression, and the residents of the neighborhoods with high economic deprivation show significant symptoms of depression and stress [21].

4.2.20 Reducing Pollution in Urban Environments

Since air pollution, water pollution, visual pollution, and excessive accumulation of waste in urban environments cause urban stress and decrease the level of mental health, reducing them, especially air pollution, whose harmful effects on mental health have been recognized [55], and trying to create a clean environment can help improve urban mental health [4]. The presence of particles such as lead, mercury, manganese, heavy metals, pesticides, and organic solvents in the air leads to many neurological effects on humans [9]. Also, pollutants such as carbon monoxide or benzene may have direct effects on the central nervous system. Infectious agents and contagious diseases such as Covid-19 and influenza are also other pollutants of urban environments that must be considered by urban planners and designers [56]. Reducing noise pollution also significantly influence people's mental well-being [57]. Light pollution, which is known as the cause of disruption in the adaptable and predictable 24-h solar cycle, is also another pollution affecting mental health [58].

4.2.21 Promoting Justice in Urban Environments

Promoting justice in urban environments in various aspects such as the distribution of resources and services may help to further promote mental health in urban areas [13]. Reforming health and social services and increasing fair access to them in the urban environment are among the effective solutions to reduce urban stress [59]. In addition, cities in developed and developing countries face increasing concentration of wealth and poverty in the concepts of uptown and downtown areas, and perceptions of injustice induced by them may lead to demotivation, alienation, and social conflict [59]. Also, living in deprived areas of the city, regardless of the individual's socio-economic status, is associated with behavioral and psychological problems in children [60].

4.2.22 Encouraging Proper Diet and Reducing Malnutrition

Dietary deficiencies, especially vitamin B12, have many effects on people's mental health [1]. Vitamin B5 is so important that it is referred to as anti-stress vitamin [61]. Improving access to healthy and affordable food will improve mental health and reduce urban stress [62].

4.2.23 Promoting Diversity in Urban Environments

A diverse urban space is an important precondition for socialization and mental health processes since it helps to acquire social skills. It also helps to develop social diversity and create an open city. While the diversity of urban space is an important factor for its vitality, current developments tend to homogenize neighborhoods. Fragmenting the city into homogeneous neighborhoods disrupts the dynamics of the city as an open system. Also, the lack of social and cultural diversity, in turn, can lead to the lack of social skills, which subsequently promotes social isolation and conflict in the city [26].

4.2.24 Implementing Urban Remediation Strategies

Urban remediation is the term used to describe therapeutic interventions at the individual and clinical levels in urban environments that have a positive impact on the process of enhancing mental health and reducing urban stress. These tactics are implemented in two general stages of evaluating urban practises and intervening, and they span three areas: urban design, urban planning, and housing policies [63]. The plan seeks to reacquaint patients with the city and its worthwhile pursuits (such as employment, leisure pursuits, volunteer work, etc.), as well as foster interpersonal relationships [63].

4.2.24.1 Appraisal of Urban Practices

It is vital to gather sufficient data to identify urban practises in order to ascertain whether entering the city is problematic or not before performing urban cleanup. The built environment, modes of transportation, and social contacts are crucial factors to assess at this time. Finally, cognitive maps are shown, which are mental representations of an urban environment that include both positive and negative important locations and allow for the restoration of urban practices [63].

4.2.24.2 Intervention

Intervention is defined as the psychoanalysis of urban psychosis, potential stressors, urban restoration resources and places, and attempts to improve the urban environment. Reducing the experience of urban stress, handling urban stress better, reducing anhedonia, and improving motivation in the city are important issues in this field [63].

Reducing the Experience of Urban Stress

Adapted Housing and Creating a Sense of Home

Housing and its characteristics such as housing type (high-rise or low-rise and type of ownership), housing area, housing quality (structural problems, amenities, physical risks, etc.), and neighborhood quality (social problems, physical problems, etc.) have all been associated with mental health and stress [9]. Housing is an important part of the city and reducing its impact on urban stress requires policies and programs to be set at the state and city levels [64]. Housing planning for low-income groups is a new approach to end the chronic homelessness of low-level people who are more likely to suffer from mental illnesses and drug abuse [65]. Also, it is effective to implement strategies of renting mixed-income housing to rich and deprived residents or constructing apartments including both privately owned and rental units in this field [14]. Also, in these buildings, the terrace plays a key role in promoting mental health [66]. If effectively implemented, the starter house policy will result in more stable housing, better community inclusion, and an improved quality of life for those who are homeless and have severe mental illnesses. Of course, patients who suffer from paranoia will be usually not comfortable in group housing [63]. The importance of the house and the sense of owning it affordably and autonomously have many effects on the recovery process of people with mental illnesses [67].

Residential stability of the neighborhood and the concentration of the elderly, regardless of indicators of economic deprivation, is an aspect of social integration that has been associated with depression and stress. The longer residents live in a neighborhood, the less likely they are to have mental health diseases, while the higher the number of elderly living in an environment, the higher the likelihood of depression symptoms [21]. In fact, migration is a risk factor for mental illnesses, including schizophrenia and stress [68] and residential mobility at all ages, especially during adolescence, has a great impact on mental health [69].

Increasing Contact with Restorative Places

It is crucial to have places that allow us to replenish ourselves in a world where there is sensory overload. These locations are referred to as tranquil or healing settings. One of the key aspects in the design of these places is comprehending the ideal interaction between hearing and sight [70]. In the context of the "GAPS" approach, urban planning and design may support mental health through these locations. The term "GAPS" stands for "green, active, pro-social, and safe places" [11]. Urban green spaces enhance traffic, traffic flow, noise pollution reduction, social engagement, and stress reduction. Positive effects on both physical and mental health can be seen in safe environments and in environments that encourage physical activity [65]. Although improving the social environment and its networks can enhance people's mental health [44] the extensive role of these areas has always been neglected [71, 72]. Table 4.1 introduces this strategy.

Art education sites and observing them have a great therapeutic effect on mental health patients, in this sense, these sites can be considered restorative places in urban environments [71, 72]. Also, recreational places, museums, places of worship [73], houses in various forms and places from which one can see landscapes [67], and places of rich historical fascination [63], places with natural sounds [74], and blue spaces such as seas, lakes, ponds, etc. also act as restorative places [75].

Table 4.1 Introduction of "GAPS" strategy in urban design [11]

GAPS	G	Green places	Green and blue spaces such as parks, forests, gardens, lakes, rivers, and seas are promising factors for improving mental health through urban design.
	A	Active places	Green spaces in the city play an important role in promoting physical activities, and exercises have a positive effect on mental health and subjective well-being. Exercises have a positive effect on depression, anxiety, and schizophrenia. Also, accessible and walkable parks and playgrounds may facilitate physical activities and need to be considered by urban designers. In addition, the availability of cycling routes and public transportation, including the subway, can reduce the use of cars, which are associated with more traffic, noise, and air pollution, and thus reduce stress.
	P	Pro-social places	Public open spaces, meeting centers, public buildings, promoting social integration and networking, as well as the structure of neighborhoods may affect social connectivity.
	S	Safe places	The crime and violence rates and perceived insecurity may affect the subjective well-being and mental health of city residents. The urban design may improve security by providing a surveillance system, determining public-private zones, providing full access to public spaces and the control of them, and avoiding isolated parks or streets that may attract criminals.

Planning and Regulating the Trajectories (Mobility) in the City

Mobility is treated as an important aspect of urban planning and active mobility in the city promotes meaningful social connections and promotes a sense of control over the environment. The later daily trips end, the more complex they are, and the more single-functional the destinations, the more stress a person experiences [26]. One important method for patients in the city to control their stress has been suggested: the mobilities of urban sidewalks and their programming. For instance, this strategy seeks to stay away from busy or noisy streets or to lessen the chance of running into familiar faces, or in other words, to make the urban environment more predictable. Regarding this, a number of projects have been created to assist in defining a path throughout the city based on several criteria, such as computing the most enjoyable, safest, or fastest route. These applications could be helpful resources for patients looking for the ideal urban walking route [63]. Also since the increase in the volume of vehicle traffic [76] and the crowding of city streets and sidewalks [77] are related to psychological distress, these tools are also effective in finding the best route in terms of traffic and population density. Another way to organize mobility is to pay attention to the rhythm of walking. People speed up their walking rhythm when they encounter sources of stress and speed down it in more favorable environmental conditions. This feature can be used in planning and regulating mobility in the city [67].

Handling Urban Stress Better

Reinforcing or Adapting Psychological and Social Tactics

People use different tactics to encounter stress in the urban environment, the most common of which is to create sensory bubbles of isolation and create an atmosphere of comfort. As the examples of sensory bubbles of isolation, one can refer to social interaction with others, the use of technologies such as headphones, immersion in thoughts, and disconnection from the environment [30]. Creating an atmosphere of comfort refers to creating places where there is the possibility of escape, places where there is a visible landscape, and places where social interactions can be strengthened [30]. Activities such as being in a cafe, shopping, walking, or sitting in a park or city street can psychologically recover persons. Of course, the presence of family or friends activates psychological recovery and lack of safety hinders the recovery process [73]. Also, the level of fatigue also influences the possibility of restoration [73] and the hometown or social background also form people's restoration preferences [73]. In fact, these tactics are different in different people and they should be appraised in patients. There is a need for further research to assess how well existing psychological and social tactics can be integrated into an urban treatment [63].

Treatment of Paranoid Ideation

Paranoia is one of the most common mental disorders that are associated with significant distress and disruption in a person's life [78]. Paranoia and mental distress increase as social stress (social failure, high population density, low ethnic density, facing violence, etc.) increases in the environment and environmental stress may play an important role in the onset and continuation of psychosis [79]. Social and economic deprivations are also other factor influencing the formation of paranoid thoughts [46], compared to staying at home, exposure to urban streets leads to a significant increase in paranoia, anxiety, stress, and negative beliefs about oneself and others, and the result of anxiety and depression induced by social exposure in urban environments is the formation of paranoid thoughts [80]. Short and small interventions in the urban environment will significantly reduce the level of distress. A research team has developed a smartphone application (SlowMo) targeting paranoid thoughts and assisting patients [63].

Go-Along Therapy

Walking can be a useful therapeutic strategy, and being accompanied by friends and family members or a therapist while walking on a safe path can significantly reduce urban stress. Some psychotic patients or those experiencing high stress due to social stigma, paranoia, etc. cannot leave the house or receive a regular treatment, and even, some are afraid of being alone. Therefore, they need the intervention of mobile teams that can accompany them to places they would fear going alone. The strategy of go-along with a therapist to face urban stressors can be used to develop coping strategies. Communication with the therapist can be virtual (communication through smartphones) or real (presence of the therapist), and the patient can be accompanied by one of his friends or relatives in the initial stages [63]. Of course, the context of walking is different in psychological recovery and rural walking or walking in green spaces without stress is more beneficial compared to urban walking [81]. Also, walking in historical fabrics and urban spaces with natural elements has many psychological benefits, while urban traffic has adverse effects [82].

Strengthening Cognitive Resources

Theoretical literature implies that cognitive deficits (thinking, concentration, learning, and memory disorders) may make a person more vulnerable to urban stress. Also, the characteristics of an urban environment (such as disorderly architecture, advertisement, traffic, noise, etc.) can promote these deficits [63]. These deficits also play a role in causing other mental problems such as schizophrenia [83]. Strengthening cognitive resources with measures such as route planning, urban transportation planning, and selective attention (a person's effort to pay attention to non-stressful items) may be useful for adapting to a stressful urban environment [63].

Reducing Anhedonia and Improving Motivation in the City

Patients with anhedonia appear to be less able than average people to derive pleasure from exposure to pleasurable environments. Because of this, group-based therapies like the Positive Emotions Programme for Schizophrenia (PEPS), which work to increase motivation and pleasure in people with schizophrenia, may be helpful in this area. In fact, it is beneficial to tailor such strategies to particular facets of city avoidance and combine them with the planning of enjoyable group activities in a city setting. Utilising modern technologies, such as ecological momentary interventions, virtual reality, and mobile applications; trauma-focused therapy; stress management practises (such as relaxation, meditation, and exercise); and fostering urban group walking are all helpful in this area [63].

4.3 Conclusion

In this chapter, after reviewing the research on urban mental health and removing the irrelevant ones, 85 research were identified to be relevant and 33 solutions were extracted from them through content analysis. Next, the frequency of each solution was investigated and their repetition percentage was determined. Table 4.2 introduces these solutions.

Reviewing international studies has identified 33 solutions in this field. "Improving the accessibility and quality of green spaces" (14.52%) is the most frequent solution, followed by the solutions of "Adapted housing and creating a sense of home" (8.06%), "Improving social interactions" (6.45%), " Increasing contact with restorative" (5.65), "Mental health-enhancing urban design", and "Promoting social support and cohesion and reducing social deprivation" (4.84%), respectively. Figure 4.3 shows the repetition percentage of each solution.

Table 4.2 Summary of solutions to reduce urban stress

Solution No.			1	2	3	4	5	6	7	8
Expert	Reference	Year	Holding mental health promotion workshops	Improving access to mental health services	Innovative approaches such as mobile health apps and online services	Improving the lighting in homes and urban spaces	Improving the accessibility and quality of green spaces	Developing and implementing a comprehensive mental health plan	Mental health-enhancing urban design	Reducing time wastage and time pressure on citizens
Lazarus and Cohen	[49]	1977								
Lewis and Sturgill	[29]	1979								
Baum et al.	[33]	1981								
McGrath	[8]	1999				*				
Freudenberg	[59]	2000								
Caracci and Enrique Mezzich	[7]	2001								
Kalff et al.	[60]	2001								
Ewart and Suchday	[53]	2002								
Evans	[2]	2003				*	*			
Semenza	[44]	2003								
Van os	[71]	2004							*	
Galea	[13]	2005							*	
Lloyd et al.	[34]	2005							*	
Miller and Phillips	[37]	2005								

De Silva	[42]	2005								
Caracci	[7]	2006		*				*		
Maas et al.	[24]	2006					*			
Fuller et al.	[10]	2007					*			
Swinnen & Selten	[38]	2007								
Caracci	[50]	2008								
Abe et al.	[55]	2008								
French	[45]	2009								
Van den Berg et al.	[19]	2010					*			
Pheasant et al.	[70]	2010								
Thoits	[40]	2011								
Roe and Aspinall	[81]	2011								
Nanda et al.	[72]	2011								
Miles et al.	[21]	2012					*			
Rishi and Khuntia	[4]	2012					*			
Beil and Hanes	[16]	2013					*			
Rodriguez and Rosas	[27]	2013								*
Bedrosian and Nelson	[58]	2013								
Sarkar et al.	[66]	2013								

(continued)

Table 4.2 (continued)

Solution No.			1	2	3	4	5	6	7	8
Expert	Reference	Year	Holding mental health promotion workshops	Improving access to mental health services	Innovative approaches such as mobile health apps and online services	Improving the lighting in homes and urban spaces	Improving the accessibility and quality of green spaces	Developing and implementing a comprehensive mental health plan	Mental health-enhancing urban design	Reducing time wastage and time pressure on citizens
Lederbogen et al.	[56]	2013								
Bertotti et al.	[43]	2013								
Alcock et al.	[12]	2014					*			
Wickham et al.	[46]	2014								
Nnebue et al.	[62]	2014								
Paksarian et al.	[69]	2015								
Gascon et al.	[75]	2015								
Freeman et al.	[80]	2015								
Adli et al.	[26]	2016							*	
Söderström et al.	[30]	2016								
Newbury et al.	[41]	2016								
Staats et al.	[73]	2016								
Veling et al.	[79]	2016								
Gong et al.	[76]	2016								
Gruebner et al.	[13]	2017					*			
Vujcic et al.	[28]	2017								
Krzywicka and Katarzyna	[74]	2017								

Söderström et al.	[67]	2017								
Toulopoulou et al.	[83]	2017								
Neale et al.	[77]	2017								
Le et al.	[84]	2017								
Knöll et al.	[32]	2017								
Hazer et al.	[17]	2018					*			
Herrera et al.	[18]	2018					*			
Castillejos et al.	[68]	2018								
Manning	[36]	2018								
Okkels et al.	[65]	2018								
Szabo	[64]	2018								
Bornioli et al.	[82]	2018								
Elsamahy and Abd El-Fattah	[3]	2018								
Cerrato and Halamka	[1]	2019			*					
Larcombe et al.	[14]	2019					*			
Joshua et al.	[48]	2019								
Abrahamyan Empson et al.	[23]	2019					*			
Didonato	[61]	2019								
Yang et al.	[20]	2019					*			
Baumann et al.	[63]	2019								

(continued)

Table 4.2 (continued)

Solution No.			1	2	3	4	5	6	7	8
Expert	Reference	Year	Holding mental health promotion workshops	Improving access to mental health services	Innovative approaches such as mobile health apps and online services	Improving the lighting in homes and urban spaces	Improving the accessibility and quality of green spaces	Developing and implementing a comprehensive mental health plan	Mental health-enhancing urban design	Reducing time wastage and time pressure on citizens
Vojnovic et al.	[47]	2019								
Neale et al.	[25]	2019					*			
Weeland et al.	[22]	2019					*			
Meloni et al.	[35]	2019								
D'Acci et al.	[15]	2020					*			*
Jevtic	[5]	2020	*	*						
Adli and Schondorf	[31]	2020							*	
Ventriglio et al.	[11]	2020					*		*	
	Repetition		1	2	1	2	18	1	6	2
	Repetition percentage		0.81	1.61	0.81	1.61	14.52	0.81	4.84	1.61

Solution No.			9	10	11	12	13	14	15	16	17
Expert	Reference	Year	Promoting urban therapeutic gardening	Controlling population density and building density	Enhancing urban resilience	Improving identity and a sense of belonging to the city	Revitalizing cultural and religious rituals	Promoting social support and reducing social deprivation	Improving social interactions	Improving the accessibility and variety of free time activities	Improving local integration
Lazarus and Cohen	[49]	1977								*	
Lewis and Sturgill	[29]	1979	*								
Baum et al.	[33]	1981			*						
McGrath	[8]	1999									
Freudenberg	[59]	2000									
Caracci and Enrique Mezzich	[7]	2001					*				
Kalff et al.	[60]	2001									
Ewart and Suchday	[53]	2002									
Evans	[2]	2003									
Semenza	[44]	2003							*		
Van os	[71]	2004							*		
Galea	[13]	2005									
Lloyd et al.	[34]	2005			*						
Miller and Phillips	[37]	2005			*	*			*		
De Silva	[42]	2005							*		

(continued)

Table 4.2 (continued)

Solution No.			9	10	11	12	13	14	15	16	17
Expert	Reference	Year	Promoting urban therapeutic gardening	Controlling population density and building density	Enhancing urban resilience	Improving identity and a sense of belonging to the city	Revitalizing cultural and religious rituals	Promoting social support and reducing social deprivation	Improving social interactions	Improving the accessibility and variety of free time activities	Improving local integration
Caracci	[7]	2006									
Maas et al.	[24]	2006									
Fuller et al.	[10]	2007									
Swinnen & Selten	[38]	2007				*					
Caracci	[50]	2008									
Abe et al.	[55]	2008									
French	[45]	2009							*		
Van den Berg et al.	[19]	2010									
Pheasant et al.	[70]	2010									
Thoits	[40]	2011						*			
Roe and Aspinall	[81]	2011									
Nanda et al.	[72]	2011									
Miles et al.	[21]	2012						*			
Rishi and Khuntia	[4]	2012						*		*	

Beil and Hanes	[16]	2013									
Rodriguez and Rosas	[27]	2013									
Bedrosian and Nelson	[58]	2013									
Sarkar et al.	[66]	2013									
Lederbogen et al.	[56]	2013									
Bertotti et al.	[43]	2013							*		
Alcock et al.	[12]	2014									
Wickham et al.	[46]	2014						*			
Nnebue et al.	[62]	2014									
Paksarian et al.	[69]	2015									
Gascon et al.	[75]	2015									
Freeman et al.	[80]	2015									
Adli et al.	[26]	2016									
Söderström et al.	[30]	2016		*							
Newbury et al.	[41]	2016						*			
Staats et al.	[73]	2016									
Veling et al.	[79]	2016									
Gong et al.	[76]	2016									

(continued)

Table 4.2 (continued)

Solution No.			9	10	11	12	13	14	15	16	17
Expert	Reference	Year	Promoting urban therapeutic gardening	Controlling population density and building density	Enhancing urban resilience	Improving identity and a sense of belonging to the city	Revitalizing cultural and religious rituals	Promoting social support and reducing social deprivation	Improving social interactions	Improving the accessibility and variety of free time activities	Improving local integration
Gruebner et al.	[13]	2017		*							
Vujcic et al.	[28]	2017	*								
Krzywicka and Katarzyna	[74]	2017									
Söderström et al.	[67]	2017									
Toulopoulou et al.	[83]	2017									
Neale et al.	[77]	2017									
Le et al.	[84]	2017									
Knöll et al.	[32]	2017		*							
Hazer et al.	[17]	2018									
Herrera et al.	[18]	2018									
Castillejos et al.	[68]	2018									
Manning	[36]	2018				*			*		
Okkels et al.	[65]	2018									
Szabo	[64]	2018									
Bornioli et al.	[82]	2018									

Elsamahy and Abd El-Fattah	[3]	2018									
Cerrato and Halamka	[1]	2019									
Larcombe et al.	[14]	2019									
Joshua et al.	[48]	2019									*
Abrahamyan Empson et al.	[23]	2019									
Didonato	[61]	2019									
Yang et al.	[20]	2019									
Baumann et al.	[63]	2019									
Vojnovic et al.	[47]	2019									*
Neale et al.	[25]	2019									
Weeland et al.	[22]	2019									
Meloni et al.	[35]	2019				*					
D'Acci et al.	[15]	2020									
Jevtic	[5]	2020									
Adli and Schondorf	[31]	2020		*	*		*	*	*		
Ventriglio et al.	[11]	2020									
	Repetition		2	5	4	4	2	6	8	2	2
	Repetition percentage		1.61	4.03	3.23	3.23	1.61	4.84	6.45	1.61	1.61

(continued)

Table 4.2 (continued)

Solution No.			18	19	20	21	22	23	24	25	26
Expert	Reference	Year	Improving people's control over the environment	Applying the principles of smart growth and new urbanism	Not using outdated styles such as modern style	Reducing economic deprivation	Reducing pollution in urban environments	Promoting justice	Encouraging proper diet and reducing malnutrition	Promoting diversity in urban environments	Adapted housing and creating a sense of home
Lazarus and Cohen	[49]	1977	*								
Lewis and Sturgill	[29]	1979									
Baum et al.	[33]	1981									
McGrath	[8]	1999									
Freudenberg	[59]	2000						*			
Caracci and Enrique Mezzich	[7]	2001									
Kalff et al.	[60]	2001				*					
Ewart and Suchday	[53]	2002				*					
Evans	[2]	2003	*				*				*
Semenza	[44]	2003									
Van os	[71]	2004									
Galea	[13]	2005									
Lloyd et al.	[34]	2005									
Miller and Phillips	[37]	2005									

De Silva	[42]	2005									
Caracci	[7]	2006									
Maas et al.	[24]	2006									
Fuller et al.	[10]	2007									
Swinnen & Selten	[38]	2007									
Caracci	[50]	2008		*							
Abe et al.	[55]	2008					*				
French	[45]	2009									
Van den Berg et al.	[19]	2010									
Pheasant et al.	[70]	2010									
Thoits	[40]	2011									
Roe and Aspinall	[81]	2011									
Nanda et al.	[72]	2011									
Miles et al.	[21]	2012		*		*					*
Rishi and Khuntia	[4]	2012			*		*				
Beil and Hanes	[16]	2013									
Rodriguez and Rosas	[27]	2013									
Bedrosian and Nelson	[58]	2013					*				
Sarkar et al.	[66]	2013									*

(continued)

Table 4.2 (continued)

Solution No.			18	19	20	21	22	23	24	25	26
Expert	Reference	Year	Improving people's control over the environment	Applying the principles of smart growth and new urbanism	Not using outdated styles such as modern style	Reducing economic deprivation	Reducing pollution in urban environments	Promoting justice	Encouraging proper diet and reducing malnutrition	Promoting diversity in urban environments	Adapted housing and creating a sense of home
Lederbogen et al.	[56]	2013					*				
Bertotti et al.	[43]	2013									
Alcock et al.	[12]	2014									
Wickham et al.	[46]	2014									
Nnebue et al.	[62]	2014							*		
Paksarian et al.	[69]	2015									*
Gascon et al.	[75]	2015									
Freeman et al.	[80]	2015									
Adli et al.	[26]	2016									
Söderström et al.	[30]	2016									
Newbury et al.	[41]	2016									
Staats et al.	[73]	2016									
Veling et al.	[79]	2016									
Gong et al.	[76]	2016									

Gruebner et al.	[13]	2017						*			
Vujcic et al.	[28]	2017									
Krzywicka and Katarzyna	[74]	2017									
Söderström et al.	[67]	2017									*
Toulopoulou et al.	[83]	2017									
Neale et al.	[77]	2017									
Le et al.	[84]	2017			*						
Knöll et al.	[32]	2017									
Hazer et al.	[17]	2018									
Herrera et al.	[18]	2018									
Castillejos et al.	[68]	2018									*
Manning	[36]	2018									
Okkels et al.	[65]	2018									*
Szabo	[64]	2018									*
Bornioli et al.	[82]	2018									
Elsamahy and Abd El-Fattah	[3]	2018		*							
Cerrato and Halamka	[1]	2019							*		
Larcombe et al.	[14]	2019									*

(continued)

Table 4.2 (continued)

Solution No.			18	19	20	21	22	23	24	25	26
Expert	Reference	Year	Improving people's control over the environment	Applying the principles of smart growth and new urbanism	Not using outdated styles such as modern style	Reducing economic deprivation	Reducing pollution in urban environments	Promoting justice	Encouraging proper diet and reducing malnutrition	Promoting diversity in urban environments	Adapted housing and creating a sense of home
Joshua et al.	[48]	2019									
Abrahamyan Empson et al.	[23]	2019									
Didonato	[61]	2019							*		
Yang et al.	[20]	2019									
Baumann et al.	[63]	2019									*
Vojnovic et al.	[47]	2019									
Neale et al.	[25]	2019									
Weeland et al.	[22]	2019									
Meloni et al.	[35]	2019									
D'Acci et al.	[15]	2020									
Jevtic	[5]	2020									
Adli and Schondorf	[31]	2020								*	
Ventriglio et al.	[11]	2020									
	Repetition		2	3	2	3	5	2	3	1	10
	Repetition percentage		1.61	2.42	1.61	2.42	4.03	1.61	2.42	0.81	8.06

Solution No.			27	28	29	30	31	32	33
Expert	Reference	Year	Increasing contact with restorative places	Planning and regulating trajectories in the city	Reinforcing or adapting psychological and social tactics	Treatment of paranoid ideation	Go-along therapy	Strengthening cognitive resources	Reducing anhedonia and improving motivation in the city
Lazarus and Cohen	[49]	1977							
Lewis and Sturgill	[29]	1979							
Baum et al.	[33]	1981							
McGrath	[8]	1999							
Freudenberg	[59]	2000							
Caracci and Enrique Mezzich	[7]	2001							
Kalff et al.	[60]	2001							
Ewart and Suchday	[53]	2002							
Evans	[2]	2003							
Semenza	[44]	2003							
Van os	[71]	2004							
Galea	[13]	2005							
Lloyd et al.	[34]	2005							
Miller and Phillips	[37]	2005							
De Silva	[42]	2005							
Caracci	[7]	2006							

(continued)

Table 4.2 (continued)

Solution No.			27	28	29	30	31	32	33
Expert	Reference	Year	Increasing contact with restorative places	Planning and regulating trajectories in the city	Reinforcing or adapting psychological and social tactics	Treatment of paranoid ideation	Go-along therapy	Strengthening cognitive resources	Reducing anhedonia and improving motivation in the city
Maas et al.	[24]	2006							
Fuller et al.	[10]	2007							
Swinnen & Selten	[38]	2007							
Caracci	[50]	2008							
Abe et al.	[55]	2008							
French	[45]	2009							
Van den Berg et al.	[19]	2010							
Pheasant et al.	[70]	2010	*						
Thoits	[40]	2011							
Roe and Aspinall	[81]	2011					*		
Nanda et al.	[72]	2011	*						
Miles et al.	[21]	2012							
Rishi and Khuntia	[4]	2012							
Beil and Hanes	[16]	2013							
Rodriguez and Rosas	[27]	2013							
Bedrosian and Nelson	[58]	2013							

Sarkar et al.	[66]	2013							
Lederbogen et al.	[56]	2013							
Bertotti et al.	[43]	2013							
Alcock et al.	[12]	2014							
Wickham et al.	[46]	2014				*			
Nnebue et al.	[62]	2014							
Paksarian et al.	[69]	2015							
Gascon et al.	[75]	2015	*						
Freeman et al.	[80]	2015				*			
Adli et al.	[26]	2016							
Söderström et al.	[30]	2016							
Newbury et al.	[41]	2016							
Staats et al.	[73]	2016	*		*				
Veling et al.	[79]	2016				*			
Gong et al.	[76]	2016		*					
Gruebner et al.	[13]	2017							
Vujcic et al.	[28]	2017							
Krzywicka and Katarzyna	[74]	2017	*						
Söderström et al.	[67]	2017		*	*				
Toulopoulou et al.	[83]	2017						*	
Neale et al.	[77]	2017		*					
Le et al.	[84]	2017							

(continued)

Table 4.2 (continued)

Solution No.			27	28	29	30	31	32	33
Expert	Reference	Year	Increasing contact with restorative places	Planning and regulating trajectories in the city	Reinforcing or adapting psychological and social tactics	Treatment of paranoid ideation	Go-along therapy	Strengthening cognitive resources	Reducing anhedonia and improving motivation in the city
Knöll et al.	[32]	2017							
Hazer et al.	[17]	2018							
Herrera et al.	[18]	2018							
Castillejos et al.	[68]	2018							
Manning	[36]	2018							
Okkels et al.	[65]	2018							
Szabo	[64]	2018							
Bornioli et al.	[82]	2018					*		
Elsamahy and Abd El-Fattah	[3]	2018							
Cerrato and Halamka	[1]	2019							
Larcombe et al.	[14]	2019							
Joshua et al.	[48]	2019							
Abrahamyan Empson et al.	[23]	2019							
Didonato	[61]	2019							
Yang et al.	[20]	2019							
Baumann et al.	[63]	2019	*	*	*	*	*	*	*
Vojnovic et al.	[47]	2019							
Neale et al.	[25]	2019							
Weeland et al.	[22]	2019							

Meloni et al.	[35]	2019							
D'Acci et al.	[15]	2020							
Jevtic	[5]	2020							
Adli and Schondorf	[31]	2020		*					
Ventriglio et al.	[11]	2020	*						
	Repetition		7	5	3	4	3	2	1
	Repetition percentage		5.65	4.03	2.42	3.23	2.42	1.61	0.81

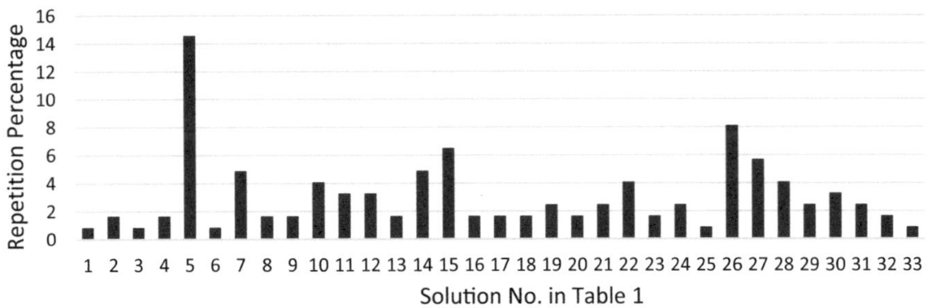

Fig. 4.3 The graph of the repetition percentage of each solution in the theoretical literature

References

1. Cerrato P, Halamk J. The transformative power of mobile medicine. Ment Health. 2019;2019:109–16. https://doi.org/10.1016/B978-0-12-814923-2.00006-4.
2. Evans BE, Buil JM, Burk WJ, Cillessen AHN, van Lier PAC. Urbanicity is associated with behavioral and emotional problems in elementary school-aged children. J Child Fam Stud. 2018;27:2193–205. https://doi.org/10.1007/s10826-018-1062z.
3. Elsamahy EM, Abd El-Fattah R. Designing non-stressed psychological public spaces. BAU J Health Well-Being. 2018;2018:121–32.
4. Rishi P, Khuntia G. Urban environmental stress and behavioral adaptation in Bhopal City of India. Urban Stud Res. 2012;2012:1–9. https://doi.org/10.1155/2012/635061.
5. Jevtic M. Building capacity for public urban mental health – example of reflecting citizens workshops. Eur J Pub Health. 2020;30:ckaa165.975. https://doi.org/10.1093/eurpub/ckaa165.975.
6. Suárez C, Machin Suárez R. Medicalisation in public primary mental health care services in Chile. Soc Theory Health. 2020;19:309–30. https://doi.org/10.1057/s41285-020-00130-4.
7. Caracci G. Urban mental health: an international survey. Int J Ment Health. 2006;35(1):39–45. https://doi.org/10.2753/imh0020-7411350103.
8. McGrath J, Saha S, Welham J, El Saadi O, MacCauley C, Chant D. A systematic review of the incidence of schizophrenia: the distribution of rates and the influence of sex, urbanicity, migrant status and methodology. BMC Med. 2014;2:13. https://doi.org/10.1186/1741-7015-2-13.
9. Evans GW. The built environment and mental health. J Urban Health. 2003;80(4):536–55. https://doi.org/10.1093/jurban/jtg063.
10. Fuller RA, Irvine KN, Devine-Wright P, Warren PH, Gaston KJ. Psychological benefits of greenspace increase with biodiversity. Biol Lett. 2007;3(4):390–4. https://doi.org/10.1098/rsbl.2007.0149.
11. Ventriglio A, Torales J, Castaldelli-Maia JM, De Berardis D, Bhugra D. Urbanization and emerging mental health issues. CNS Spectr. 2020;2020:1–8. https://doi.org/10.1017/S1092852920001236.
12. Alcock I, White MP, Wheeler BW, Fleming LE, Depledge MH. Longitudinal effects on mental health of moving to greener and less green urban areas. Environ Sci Technol. 2014;48(2):1247–55. https://doi.org/10.1021/es403688w.
13. Gruebner O, Rapp MA, Adli M, Kluge U, Galea S, Heinz A. Cities and mental health. Dtsch Arztebl Int. 2017;114:121–7. https://doi.org/10.3238/arztebl.2017.0121.
14. Larcombe E, Logan P, Horwitz A. High-rise apartments and urban mental Health—historical and contemporary views. Challenges. 2019;10(2):34. https://doi.org/10.3390/challe10020034.

15. D'Acci LS. Urbanicity mental costs valuation: a review and urban-societal planning consideration. Mind Soc. 2020;9:223–35. https://doi.org/10.1007/s11299-020-00235-3.
16. Beil K, Hanes D. The influence of urban natural and built environments on physiological and psychological measures of stress: a pilot study. Int J Environ Res Public Health. 2013;10:1250–67. https://doi.org/10.3390/ijerph10041250.
17. Hazer M, Formica MK, Dieterlen S, Morley CP. The relationship between self-reported exposure to greenspace and human stress in Baltimore, MD. Landsc Urban Plan. 2018;169:47–56. https://doi.org/10.1016/j.landurbplan.2017.08.006.
18. Herrera R, Markevych I, Berger U, Genuneit J, Gerlich J, Nowak D, et al. Greenness and job-related chronic stress in young adults: a prospective cohort study in Germany. BMJ Open. 2018;8(6):e021599. https://doi.org/10.1136/bmjopen-2018-021599.
19. van den Berg AE, Maas J, Verheij RA, Groenewegen PP. Green space as a buffer between stressful life events and health. Soc Sci Med. 2010;70(8):1203–10. https://doi.org/10.1016/j.socscimed.2010.01.002.
20. Yang T, Barnett R, Fan Y, Li L. The effect of urban green space on uncertainty stress and life stress: a nationwide study of university students in China. Health Place. 2019;59:102199. https://doi.org/10.1016/j.healthplace.2019.102199.
21. Miles R, Coutts C, Mohamadi A. Neighborhood urban form, social environment, and depression. J Urban Health. 2012;89(1):1–18. https://doi.org/10.1007/s11524-011-9621-2.
22. Weeland J, Laceulle OM, Nederhof E, Overbeek G, Reijneveld SA. The greener the better? Does neighborhood greenness buffer the effects of stressful life events on externalizing behavior in late adolescence? Health Place. 2019;58:102163. https://doi.org/10.1016/j.healthplace.2019.102163.
23. Abrahamyan Empson L, Baumann PS, Söderström O, Codeluppi Z, Söderström D, Conus P. Urbanicity: the need for new avenues to explore the link between urban living and psychosis. Early Interv Psychiatry. 2020;14(4):398–409. https://doi.org/10.1111/eip.12861.
24. Maas J, Verheij RA, Groenewegen P, de Vries S, Spreeuwenberg P. Green space, urbanity, and health: how strong is the relation? J Epidemiol Commun Health. 2006;60(7):587–92. https://doi.org/10.1136/jech.2005.043125.
25. Neale C, Aspinall P, Roe J, Tilley S, Mavros P, Cinderby S, et al. The impact of walking in different urban environments on brain activity in older people. Cities Health. 2019;4:94–106. https://doi.org/10.1080/23748834.2019.1619893.
26. Adli M, Berger M, Brakemeier E-L, Engel L, Fingerhut J, Hehl R, et al. Neurourbanistik – ein methodischer Schulterschluss zwischen Stadtplanung und Neurowissenschaften. Die Psychiatrie. 2016;13:70–8.
27. Rodríguez MD, Rosas CMC. Ambient urban games for reducing the stress of commuters crossing the Mexico-US border. In: Urzaiz G, Ochoa SF, Bravo J, Chen LL, Oliveira J, editors. Ubiquitous computing and ambient intelligence. Context-awareness and context-driven interaction, Lecture notes in computer science, vol. 8276. Cham: Springer; 2013. https://doi.org/10.1007/978-3-319-03176-7_52.
28. Vujcic M, Tomicevic-Dubljevic J, Grbic M, Lecic-Tosevski D, Vukovic O, Toskovic O. Nature based solution for improving mental health and well-being in urban areas. Environ Res. 2017;158:385–92. https://doi.org/10.1016/j.envres.2017.06.030.
29. Lewis CA, Sturgill S. Comment: Healing in the urban environment a person/plant viewpoint. J Am Plann Assoc. 1979;45(3):330–8. https://doi.org/10.1080/01944367908976971.
30. Söderström O, Empson LA, Codeluppi Z, Söderström D, Baumann PS, Conus P. Unpacking 'the City': an experience-based approach to the role of urban living in psychosis. Health Place. 2016;42:104–10. https://doi.org/10.1016/j.healthplace.2016.09.002.
31. Adli M, Schondorf J. Macht uns die Stadt krank. Wirkung von Stadtstress auf Emotionen, Verhalten und psychische Gesundheit; Does the city make us ill? The effect of urban stress on emotions, behavior, and mental health. Bundesgesundheitsbl. 2020;63:979–86. https://doi.org/10.1007/s00103-020-03185-w.

32. Knöll M, Neuheuser K, Cleff T, Rudolph-Cleff A. A tool to predict perceived urban stress in open public spaces. Environ Plan B Urban Anal City Sci. 2017;45:797–813. https://doi.org/10.1177/0265813516686971.
33. Baum AS, Jerome EB, Carlene S. Stress and the environment. Soc Issues. 1981;37(1):4–35. https://doi.org/10.1111/j.1540-4560.1981.tb01056.x.
34. Lloyd S, Kelly R, Kimberly G, Joshua R. Challenges of urban mental health disaster planning. J Aggress Maltreat Trauma. 2005;10(3):695–706. https://doi.org/10.1300/J146v10n03_03.
35. Meloni A, Fornara F, Carrus G. Predicting pro-environmental behaviors in the urban context: the direct or moderated effect of urban stress, city identity, and worldviews. Cities. 2019;88:83–90. https://doi.org/10.1016/j.cities.2019.01.001.
36. Manning N. Sociology, biology and mechanisms in urban mental health. Soc Theory Health. 2018;17:1–22. https://doi.org/10.1057/s41285-018-00085-7.
37. Miller KM, Phillips MH. Correlates of urban stress and mental health: the impact of social context on resilience. J Soc Distress Homeless. 2005;14(1–2):46–64. https://doi.org/10.1179/105307805807066301.
38. Swinnen SGHA, Selten J-P. Mood disorders and migration: meta-analysis. Br J Psychiatry. 2007;190(1):6–10. https://doi.org/10.1192/bjp.bp.105.020800.
39. Caracci G, Enrique MJ. Culture and urban mental health. Psychiatr Clin North Am. 2001;24(3):581–93. https://doi.org/10.1016/S0193-953X(05)70249-5.
40. Thoits PA. Mechanisms linking social ties and support to physical and mental health. J Health Soc Behav. 2011;52(2):145–61. https://doi.org/10.1177/0022146510395592.
41. Newbury J, Arseneault L, Caspi A, Moffitt TE, Odgers CL, Fisher HL. Why are children in urban neighborhoods at increased risk for psychotic symptoms? Findings from a UK longitudinal cohort study. Schizophr Bull. 2016;42(6):1372–83. https://doi.org/10.1093/schbul/sbw052.
42. De Silva MJ. Social capital and mental illness: a systematic review. J Epidemiol Commun Health. 2005;59(8):619–27. https://doi.org/10.1136/jech.2004.029678.
43. Bertotti M, Watts P, Netuveli G, Yu G, Schmidt E, et al. Types of social capital and mental disorder in deprived urban areas: a multilevel study of 40 disadvantaged London neighbourhoods. PLoS One. 2013;8(12):e80127. https://doi.org/10.1371/journal.pone.0080127.
44. Semenza JC. The intersection of urban planning, art, and public Health: the Sunnyside piazza. Am J Public Health. 2003;93(9):1439–41. https://doi.org/10.2105/ajph.93.9.1439.
45. French D. Residential segregation and health in Northern Ireland. Health Place. 2009;15(3):888–96. https://doi.org/10.1016/j.healthplace.2009.02.012.
46. Wickham S, Taylor P, Shevlin M, Bentall RP. The impact of social deprivation on paranoia, hallucinations, mania and depression: the role of discrimination social support, stress and trust. PLoS One. 2014;9(8):e105140. https://doi.org/10.1371/journal.pone.0105140.
47. Vojnovic I, Pearson A, Asiki G, Allen A, DeVerteuil G. Handbook of global urban health. 1st ed. Routledge; 2019. https://doi.org/10.4324/9781315465456.
48. Joshua CF, Freeman C, Bazargan-Hejazi S. Environmental interventions for physical and mental health: challenges and opportunities for Greater Los Angeles. Int J Environ Res Public Health. 2019;16(12):2180. https://doi.org/10.3390/ijerph16122180.
49. Lazarus RS, Cohen JB. Environmental stress. Hum Behav Environ. 1977;1977:89–127. https://doi.org/10.1007/978-1-4684-0808-9_3.
50. Caracci G. General concepts of the relationship between urban areas and mental health. Curr Opin Psychiatry. 2008;21(4):385–90. https://doi.org/10.1097/yco.0b013e328303e198.
51. Li J, Rose N. Urban social exclusion and mental health of China's rural-urban migrants – a review and call for research. Health Place. 2017;48:20–30. https://doi.org/10.1016/j.healthplace.2017.08.009.
52. Dye C. Health and urban living. Science. 2008;319(5864):766–9. https://doi.org/10.1126/science.1150198.
53. Ewart CK, Suchday S. Discovering how urban poverty and violence affect health: development and validation of a neighborhood stress index. Health Psychol. 2002;21(3):254–62. https://doi.org/10.1037/0278-6133.21.3.254.

54. Kluge U, Rapp MA, Mehran N, Jumaa J, Aichberger MC. Armut, migration und psychische gesundheit; Poverty, migration and mental health. Nervenarzt. 2019;90:1103–8. https://doi.org/10.1007/s00115-019-00790-2.
55. Abe KK, Brandao LDC, Tufik S, Saldiva PHN, D'Almeida V. The impact of urban air pollution exposure on the development of alterations on oxidative stress and behavioral parameters in adult mice. Ann General Psychiatry. 2008;7:S132. https://doi.org/10.1186/1744-859X-7-S1-S132.
56. Lederbogen F, Haddad L, Meyer-Lindenberg A. Urban social stress – risk factor for mental disorders. The case of schizophrenia. Environ Pollut. 2013;183:2–6. https://doi.org/10.1016/j.envpol.2013.05.046.
57. Evans GW, Wells NM, Moch A. Housing and mental health: a review of the evidence and a methodological and conceptual critique. J Soc Issues. 2003;59(3):475–500. https://doi.org/10.1111/1540-4560.00074.
58. Bedrosian TA, Nelson RJ. Influence of the modern light environment on mood. Mol Psychiatry. 2013;18(7):751–7. https://doi.org/10.1038/mp.2013.70.
59. Freudenberg N. Health promotion in the city: a review of current practice and future prospects in the United States. Annu Rev Public Health. 2000;21(1):473–503. https://doi.org/10.1146/annurev.publhealth.21.1.473.
60. Kalff AC, Kroes M, Vles JS, Hendriksen JG, Feron FJ, Steyaert J, et al. Neighbourhood level and individual level SES effects on child problem behaviour: a multilevel analysis. J Epidemiol Commun Health. 2001;55(4):246–50. https://doi.org/10.1136/jech.55.4.246.
61. Didonato. Best vitamins for stress. 2019. http://www.personanutrition.com. Accessed 7 Oct 2021.
62. Nnebue CC, Adinma ED, Queencallista N. Urbanization and health. Orient J Med. 2014;26:1–2.
63. Baumann PS, Söderström O, Abrahamyan Empson L, Söderström D, Codeluppi Z, Golay P, et al. Urban remediation: a new recovery-oriented strategy to manage urban stress after first-episode psychosis. Soc Psychiatry Psychiatr Epidemiol. 2019;55:273–83. https://doi.org/10.1007/s00127-019-01795-7.
64. Szabo CP. Urbanization and mental health. Curr Opin Psychiatry. 2018;31:256–7. https://doi.org/10.1097/YCO.0000000000000414.
65. Okkels N, Kristiansen CB, Munk-Jørgensen P, Sartorius N. Urban mental health. Curr Opin Psychiatry. 2018;31:258–64. https://doi.org/10.1097/YCO.0000000000000413.
66. Sarkar C, Gallacher J, Webster C. Urban built environment configuration and psychological distress in older men: results from the Caerphilly study. BMC Public Health. 2013;13:695. https://doi.org/10.1186/1471-2458-13-695.
67. Söderström O, Söderström D, Codeluppi Z, Abrahamyan Empson L, Conus P. Emplacing recovery: how persons diagnosed with psychosis handle stress in cities. Psychosis. 2017;9:322–9. https://doi.org/10.1080/17522439.2017.1344296.
68. Castillejos MC, Martín-Pérez C, Moreno-Küstner B. A systematic review and meta-analysis of the incidence of psychotic disorders: the distribution of rates and the influence of gender, urbanicity, immigration and socio-economic level. Psychol Med. 2018;48:2101–15. https://doi.org/10.1017/S0033291718000235.
69. Paksarian D, Eaton WW, Mortensen PB, Pedersen CB. Childhood residential mobility, schizophrenia, and bipolar disorder: a population-based study in Denmark. Schizophr Bull. 2015;41(2):346–54. https://doi.org/10.1093/schbul/sbu074.
70. Pheasant RJ, Fisher MN, Watts GR, Whitaker DJ, Horoshenkov KV. The importance of auditory-visual interaction in the construction of 'tranquil space'. J Environ Psychol. 2010;30(4):501–9. https://doi.org/10.1016/j.jenvp.2010.03.006.
71. Van Os J. Does the urban environment cause psychosis? Br J Psychiatry. 2004;184(4):287–8. https://doi.org/10.1192/bjp.184.4.287.
72. Nanda UE, Zadeh S, Owen D. Effect of visual art on patient anxiety and agitation in a mental health facility and implications for the business case. J Psychiatr Ment Health Nurs. 2011;18(5):386–93. https://doi.org/10.1111/j.1365-2850.2010.01682.x.

73. Staats H, Jahncke H, Herzog TR, Hartig T, Nater UM. Urban options for psychological restoration: common strategies in everyday situations. PLoS One. 2016;11(1):e0146213. https://doi.org/10.1371/journal.pone.0146213.
74. Krzywicka P, Byrka K. Restorative qualities of and preference for natural and urban soundscapes. Front Psychol. 2017;8:1705. https://doi.org/10.3389/fpsyg.2017.01705.
75. Gascon M, Triguero-Mas M, Martínez D, Dadvand P, Forns J, Plasència A, et al. Mental health benefits of long-term exposure to residential green and blue spaces: a systematic review. Int J Environ Res Public Health. 2015;12(4):4354–79. https://doi.org/10.3390/ijerph120404354.
76. Gong Y, Palmer S, Gallacher J, Marsden T, Fone D. A systematic review of the relationship between objective measurements of the urban environment and psychological distress. Environ Int. 2016;96:48–57. https://doi.org/10.1016/j.envint.2016.08.019.
77. Neale C, Aspinall P, Roe J, Tilley S, Mavros P, Cinderby S, et al. The aging urban brain: analyzing outdoor physical activity using the Emotiv Affectiv suite in older people. J Urban Health. 2017;94:869–80. https://doi.org/10.1007/s11524-017-0191-9.
78. Garety PA, Ward T, Freeman D, Fowler D, Emsley R, Dunn G, et al. SlowMo, a digital therapy targeting reasoning in paranoia, versus treatment as usual in the treatment of people who fear harm from others: study protocol for a randomised controlled trial. Trials. 2017;18(1):510. https://doi.org/10.1186/s13063-017-2242-7.
79. Veling W, Pot-Kolder R, Counotte J, van Os J, van der Gaag M. Environmental social stress, paranoia and psychosis liability: a virtual reality study. Schizophr Bull. 2016;2016:1363–71. https://doi.org/10.1093/schbul/sbw031.
80. Freeman D, Emsley R, Dunn G, Fowler D, Bebbington P, Kuipers E, et al. The stress of the street for patients with persecutory delusions: a test of the symptomatic and psychological effects of going outside into a busy urban area. Schizophr Bull. 2015;41(4):971–9. https://doi.org/10.1093/schbul/sbu173.
81. Roe J, Aspinall P. The restorative benefits of walking in urban and rural settings in adults with good and poor mental health. Health Place. 2011;17(1):103–13. https://doi.org/10.1016/j.healthplace.2010.09.003.
82. Bornioli A, Parkhurst G, Morgan PL. Psychological wellbeing benefits of simulated exposure to five urban settings: an experimental study from the pedestrian's perspective. J Transp Health. 2018;2018:S2214140517306977–116. https://doi.org/10.1016/j.jth.2018.02.003.
83. Toulopoulou T, Picchioni M, Mortensen PB, Petersen L. IQ, the urban environment, and their impact on future schizophrenia risk in men. Schizophr Bull. 2017;43(5):1056–63. https://doi.org/10.1093/schbul/sbw147.
84. Le TD, Payne J, Clarke C, Kelly MA, Prudenziati F, Armsby E, Penacchio O, Wilkins AJ. Discomfort from urban scenes: metabolic consequences. Landsc Urban Plan. 2017;160:61–8. https://doi.org/10.1016/j.landurbplan.2016.12.003.

Chapter 5
Identification of Urban Stress Measurement Methods

Abstract In this chapter, first, stress and urban stress measurement methods are introduced generally, and then the studies on urban stress are reviewed. Finally, the methods used in these studies are summarized to select the best urban stress measurement method.

It is still difficult to measure stress objectively. Many existing tools used for measuring psychological distress, due to clinical reasons, focus on general health outcomes, depression, or anxiety (Vojnovic et al., Handbook of global urban health, 1st ed, Routledge, 269, 2019). To measure stress, it is required to consider its type, extent, intensity, duration, onset, and frequency (Cappon, CMA J 16(8):9, 1977). Therefore, relevant physiological signals such as heart rate variability (HRV), galvanic skin response (GSR), skin temperature (ST), electroencephalogram (EEG), electrocardiogram (ECG), blood volume pulse (BVP), are considered reliable stress indicators (Kyriakou and Resch, Adv Cartogr GIScience Int Cartogr Assoc 2:1, 2019).

To measure urban stress, it is required to assess urban spaces. Even today, the advantages of biosensors, including the absence of bias, the possibility of continuous measurement with high time resolution, reducing the burden on the participants, the possibility of collecting extensive longitudinal data, and higher ecological validity than experimental studies, make these sensors the basis of stress measurement approaches in urban areas. Of course, there are numerous approaches to detect stress through physiological sensors.

It is effective to use a combination of all methods in the field of urban stress and their combination is the best option. In fact, the best urban stress measurement method is to combine the following methods: equipping places or subjects with devices such as biosensing, using applications with the capability of georeferencing data, using personal opinions of people, and interviewing people suffering from stress and mental illnesses.

Keywords Environmental stress · Urban stress · Mental health · Biosensors · Physiological signals

S. Jalilisadrabad et al., *Stress Relief Urban Planning*,
https://doi.org/10.1007/978-981-99-4202-2_5

5.1 Introduction

In this chapter, first, stress and urban stress measurement methods are introduced generally, and then the studies on urban stress are reviewed. Finally, the methods used in these studies are summarized to select the best urban stress measurement method.

5.2 Stress Measurement Methods and Tools

It is still difficult to measure stress objectively. Many existing tools used for measuring psychological distress, due to clinical reasons, focus on general health outcomes, depression, or anxiety [1]. To measure stress, it is required to consider its type, extent, intensity, duration, onset, and frequency [2]. Therefore, relevant physiological signals such as heart rate variability[1] (HRV), galvanic skin response[2] (GSR), skin temperature (ST), electroencephalogram (EEG), electrocardiogram (ECG), blood volume pulse (BVP), are considered reliable stress indicators [4]. Of course, several researchers have used a combination of these physiological signals to measure stress [4]. Electrodermal activity (EDA[3]) or galvanic skin response is the most reliable parameter for measuring emotions such as stress [5]. Another biomarker used to measure stress is the level of cortisol, which is also called the stress hormone, which is not easily applicable to measure stress caused by exposure to the environment or the city, and it must be measured in a laboratory environment [6].

Psychological stress data can be collected using a questionnaire. Perceived Stress Scale (PSS), Social Readjustment Rating Scale (SRSS), NASA Task Load Index (NASA-TLX), Self Assessment Manikin,[4] and Positive and Negative Affect Schedule (PANAS) are widely used questionnaires for measuring stress in the laboratory and daily life stress [8]. Among other stress measurement tools, we can

[1] It refers to changes in the time intervals between consecutive heartbeats, which are also called interbeat intervals (*IBIs*). Lower levels of HRV are associated with emotions such as anger, anxiety, fear, and psychological stress, and higher levels of HRV are associated with relaxation [3].

[2] It is also called electrodermal activity (EDA). It refers to the variation in the electrical properties of the skin. When a person is stimulated, the sympathetic nervous system intensify sweating, which in turn increases the conductance of the skin. So, higher levels of EDA are associated with psychological stress [3].

[3] It is also called galvanic skin response. It refers to the variation in the electrical properties of the skin. When a person is stimulated, the sympathetic nervous system intensify sweating, which in turn increases the conductance of the skin. So, higher levels of EDA are associated with psychological stress [3].

[4] It is a pictorial questionnaire that was developed to measure emotional responses such as pleasure, perceived arousal, and perceptions of dominance [7].

mention the Ecological Momentary Assessment[5] (EMA) system that can be run on smartphones. The system displays random questionnaires throughout the day and is suitable for real-life data collection. Combining data from this system and smart wristbands such as "Empatica Band" or "Microsoft Band" brings high reliability [10]. Also, Lee et al. [11] have developed a stress measurement system called Personal Digital Assistance to estimate the level of stress using physiological signals. This system detects stress by measuring heart rate, variations in skin temperature, and electrodermal activity without any discomfort through the finger and can be used as a PDA and smartphone [11].

5.3 Urban Stress Measurement Methods

To measure urban stress, it is required to assess urban spaces. Humans always perceive and assess the environment emotionally, and their emotional responses affect their daily behavior and decision-making in space [12]. The cognitive representation of urban space was started with the term "mental image" by Lynch (1960) [4]. But the first operational tool to measure urban stress was introduced by Holmes and Rahe (1977) and later developed by others [13]. The Environmental Stress Index (ZPG) was then used in 1988 to assess urban stress in 192 American communities. Population change, crowding, education, violent crime, community and individual economies, births, air quality, hazardous waste, water, and sewage were all factors included in this test, but both its conceptual and methodological criteria were inadequate. One of the errors of this test was the equal weights of factors, causing it to be greatly criticized [14]. Even today, the advantages of biosensors, including the absence of bias, the possibility of continuous measurement with high time resolution, reducing the burden on the participants, the possibility of collecting extensive longitudinal data, and higher ecological validity than experimental studies, make these sensors the basis of stress measurement approaches in urban areas [3]. Of course, there are numerous approaches to detect stress through physiological sensors, which are placed under two categories: laboratory conditions and real-world conditions [15].

Today, biosensing refers to the application of technology to gather physiological or biometric data linked to psychometric data, which is frequently examined using psychophysiological models. This technique shares many characteristics with momentary evaluation, which has a longer history in psychology. With the goal of mapping human emotional data and emotional processes to create smart technologies and algorithms capable of assessing and enhancing subjective well-being in smart cities, biosensing technology is essential to the possible usage of predictive

[5] It relies on a smartphone app that randomly alerts the user at times determined by the assessor. Then, notifications are displayed on the mobile to notify the user to complete the assessment questions. This approach minimizes the problem of biases from the past, enables real-world investigation, and increases ecological validity [9].

analytics and empathetic artificial intelligence. For instantaneous stress evaluation or biosensing, a number of techniques have been utilised, such as monitoring salivary cortisol levels, wearing biosensors on the wrist, and wearing heart rate monitors on the chest. In order to pinpoint the causal connections between the environment, the body, the brain, the mind, and behavior, ambulatory psychophysiological research techniques are also recommended. One can think of the combination of GIScience, subjective perceptions of emotions, and physiological data as different approaches to researching urban stress [6]. Rapidly developing disciplines like social networking, virtual reality, and best route finding may present interesting opportunities for stress measurement and the design of therapies to aid patients in learning new techniques and strategies. In addition, patients may benefit from using virtual reality to manage difficult social interactions [16]. The following presents numerous significant studies in this area and their methodologies:

1. Reynolds used somatic complaints, which are the most adaptive form of internalizing distress in the field of urban stress, to measure the urban stress of young people. IExpressingdistress through physical symptoms may be more supported than that psychological symptom [17].
2. Nold employed physiological signals in conjunction with GPS data in his biomapping study to identify the moods of his subjects. He gathered GSR and ST using a "biomapping device" created for this research and then turned the gathered physiological signals into maps of emotional arousal while taking into account their locations [18].
3. Bergner et al. [19] evaluated urban stress in three cities (Mannheim, Kaiserslautern, and Alexandria) in Germany and Egypt. Seven individuals who were outfitted with cameras, GPS trackers, and smart wristbands performed this measurement. The researchers used the "Stress Phase Identifier" programme to analyse the data they had gathered, and they used point density analysis to depict the urban stress spots as a "heat map of stress points" [19]. For accurate statistical conclusions, this study's sample size is too small [19]. However, efficient techniques and instruments have been applied to locate stress hotspots.
4. Huang and Gartner suggested a mobile crowdsourcing strategy in their EmoMap project to gather people's affective responses via smartphones. They created a model called Affect-Space that could be used in an Android mobile application. Users were asked to rate their "levels of comfort" in their current environment using a seven-point Likert scale (from uncomfortable (1) to comfortable (7)), with the option to also rate the environment's attractiveness, diversity, safety, and comfort [20].
5. Zeile et al. [5] looked at the tension points noted by city bikers in the Californian San Francisco Bay Area. Twelve volunteers were given a Zephyr Bioharness chest belt to measure ECG, a smart band to collect GSR, smartphones with a dedicated app to collect participant feedback, and action cameras. Physiological variables like the electrocardiogram, skin conductance, skin temperature, and heart rate variability were analysed to pinpoint stressful moments. The idea that stress causes an increase in skin conductance and a reduction in skin temperature

led to the identification of stress. To identify the causes of emotional arousal, the scientists developed stress hot spot maps and compared them with the recorded films [5].

6. Fathullah and Willis [21] recorded the GSR and movement path of participants (N = 9) during a walking route in the city of Plymouth. Then, the peaks of GSR were examined to detect stressful areas and considered stress peaks [21].
7. Chrisinger and King measured the environmental stress in a site in San Francisco using the combination of sensory data from a smart wristband (Empatica E4) and photos and audio narratives sent by citizens, and have identified the points with high or low stress [22].
8. Kyriakou and Resch [4] used physiological data (GSR and ST) obtained by the wearable sensor "Empatica E4" to study the stress on the sidewalks in the cities of Salzburg, Austria, and Cologne, Germany. Through the sensor, the individuals' subjectively experienced physiological and emotional data were captured and wirelessly transmitted to the smartphone app "eDiary." This programme tracks stressful occasions in three steps: First, based on the findings of earlier research, several criteria for stress detection and threshold values are specified. Second, the values are adjusted to accurately identify stressful periods. Third, a ternary scoring method is used to identify stressed hot and cold regions (0, 0.5, and 1). After a walk, individuals may be invited to complete a questionnaire or enter sensor data into an eDiary app on their smartphone [4].
9. Werner et al. [23] developed an interactive web map that shows the chosen route and the participants' noted locations of high stress. Each stressed node's radius in this study was 20 m. Based on an increase in skin conductance for at least 2 s and a subsequent drop in skin temperature within 5 s, stress was identified. Although the stress measured and reported on each path demonstrated a clear connection among individuals, this method results in a substantial divergence of the stress range between the participants. As a result, the method described here may typically be used to measure the perception of stress [23].
10. Neale et al. [24] equipped several elderly people with an EEG device to measure their positive (relaxation) and negative (uncomfortable) emotions while walking on three example sidewalks in London [24].
11. Teixeira et al. [25] used a smart wristband and voice sensors to measure the stress of cyclists on the cycling paths in the cities of Oxford and London (UK) and Amsterdam, Hooten, and Groningen (Netherlands). Their findings indicated the possibility of higher stress in streets shared with cars, in streets without bicycle lanes, at intersections, on poor-quality surfaces, in two-way streets, and noisy areas [25].
12. In order to understand the embodied emotional experiences of urban life, Peykett et al. (2020) looked at the possibilities of an interdisciplinary research approach and the use of citizen science approaches. With the help of biosensing (an Empatica wristband), a paper activity diary that tracked the participant's activities, two stress- and well-being-related questionnaires (the WHOQOL BREF questionnaire and the Perceived Stress Scale (PSS)), and in-depth interviews with 31 University of Birmingham (UK) and Salzburg (Austria)

employees, this study sought to identify the psychophysiological traits and stressful experiences. Urban stress is addressed using citizen science strategies that combine physiological viewpoints with those from the social sciences and humanities. Even though the use of wearable sensors opens up new opportunities for gathering data from a large number of participants, it also raises new theoretical, moral, and practical questions about how these sensors are created from a critical social science perspective and how they facilitate citizen engagement and participation. The first step in developing citizen science approaches where data protection, security, and ownership are prioritised and collaborative commitments are made is to address the ethical issues raised by the research regarding the use of wearable biosensor technology [6].

13. Versey [26] provided an overview of a mobile-phone-based go-along therapy method that can be used with a variety of other technologies and complementary methods to better understand how people respond to places and environmental stimuli. This research aimed to create a bridge between places and mental health. This research has used qualitative methods such as photovoice, in which participants were asked to capture the photos of those places stimulating them, and pod walking, which is an interactive process including digital tools (such as phone cameras, video, and blogging) to create the life story of the participants and the participants themselves usually make, edit, and analyze the videos. The final result of these methods included narrative cartographic maps [26].
14. In 2021, another study entitled "Space-time analytics of human physiology for urban planning" in the Netherlands examined 12 cyclists in terms of the relationship between the emotional arousal of cyclists (skin conductance response) and visual stimuli from the environment (the extent of visible land cover). In addition, the findings are greatly useful for the design of cycling infrastructure [27].
15. Camara et al. [28] conducted a study to measure emotions such as stress, happiness, etc. in the city of Curitiba. This research collected collaborative emotional maps through volunteers' geographic information. By showing emotions on the maps through emojis (as presented in Fig. 5.1), it emphasized that a valid way to show emotions is to integrate a modern language into maps. This research encourages a citizen-centered perspective [28].
16. On September 5, 2021, the interdisciplinary forum Neurourbanistik completed the "Your Emotional City" project in the city of Berlin. In this project, citizens were asked to mark and specify stressful points or calming points on analog maps. This project is based on citizen science and considers citizens as good experts who can transmit valuable data within a short period [29].

As stated mentioned in the studies above, different methods have been used to measure urban stress. Exploring patients' personal experiences is also another effective method in this field [30]. Online questionnaires are another method used to measure stress, in which people identify stressful places according to their memories [31]. However, researchers are still trying to better understand the specific environmental

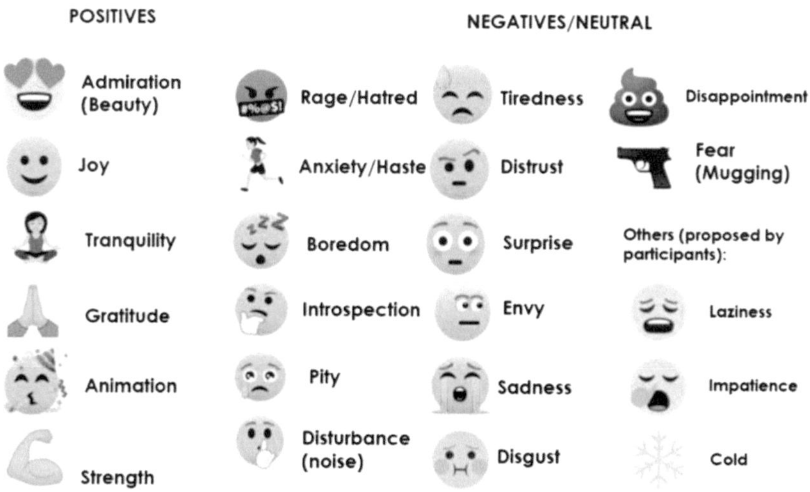

Fig. 5.1 The introduction of emojis showing emotions in the form of positives and negatives [28]

elements causing urban stress. Therefore, they are looking for methods and tools helping to more objectively examine the momentary exposure to the environment and its impact on mental health and stress [3]. What is very important in these methods is maintaining the privacy of the participants at every stage of the research process, informing them of the essential elements of the research such as the purpose, procedures, the research field, etc., and storing the data anonymously [6]. According to the studies conducted in this field and considering the effectiveness of other factors in measuring biological parameters, relying on citizen science seems to be the best and most effective method in measuring urban stress.

5.4 Conclusion

In this section, Table 5.1 summarizes different methods used for measuring urban stress according to previous studies.

According to Table 5.1 and the advantages and disadvantages of the used methods, it seems that the hybrid methods are the best urban stress measurement methods. It should be noted that there is a possibility of the influence of other conditions or issues not related to the field of cities and urbanization in all cases to some extent, because people may always assess an urban environment as stressful due to their unpleasant feelings about color, sound, environment, etc., which are rooted in their memories. This problem exists even in the evaluation of physiological signals using biosensing or new methods such as photovoice and pod walking. So, people's personal opinions are of great importance and it is better to pay attention to them along with the use of other methods. However, sometimes, people don't express their real

Table 5.1 Summary of the methods used for measuring urban stress

	Used method	Reference	Year	Advantages	Disadvantages
1	Somatic complaints	Reynolds et al. [17]	2001	The possibility of reporting the tests out of time	Unknownness of the cause of stress
2	GSR and ST physiological signals conjugated with GPS data	Nold [18]	2009	Georeferenced data	The possibility of the influence of other conditions
3	Cameras, GPS trackers, and smart wristbands	Bergner et al. [19]	2013	Georeferenced data	The small number of samples—the possibility of the influence of other conditions
4	Assessing the level of stress based on a 7-point Likert scale through an Android application	Huang and Gartner	2016	Georeferenced data- the possibility of the participation of more people	The possibility of the influence of other conditions
5	A Zephyr Bioharness chest belt (to measure ECG), a smart band (to collect GSR), smartphones with a specific app for receiving participant feedback, and action cameras	Zeile et al. [20]	2016	Georeferenced data- the possibility of the participation of more people	The small number of samples—the possibility of the influence of other conditions
6	Recording the GSR and the movement path of the participants during a walking tour	Fethullah and Willis [21]	2018	Georeferenced data	The possibility of the influence of other conditions
7	Combining sensory data from a smart wristband (Empatica E4) and photos and audio narratives sent by citizens	Chrisinger and King [22]	2018	Georeferenced data- the possibility of the participation of more people	The possibility of the influence of other conditions
8	Physiological signals (GSR and ST) and emotions that are subjectively perceived by the subjects	Kyriakou and Resch [4]	2019	Georeferenced data- the possibility of the participation of more people	The possibility of the influence of other conditions
9	An interactive web map displaying the selected route and the spots of high stress marked by the participants	Werner et al. [23]	2019	Georeferenced data-involving people's personal opinions—the possibility of participation of more people	The possibility of the influence of other conditions
10	Equipping sidewalks with an EEG device	Neale et al. [24]	2019	Georeferenced data—the possibility of the participation of more people	The possibility of the influence of other conditions

Table 5.1 (continued)

	Used method	Reference	Year	Advantages	Disadvantages
11	Exploring patients' experiences	Abrahamyan Empson et al. [30]	2019	Identification of stressful places from the point of view of patients	Non-georeferenced data
12	A smart wristband and voice sensors	Teixeira et al. [25]	2020	Georeferenced data	The possibility of the influence of other conditions
13	Biosensing (Empatica wristband), paper activity diary (which tracked the participant's activities), two questionnaires focusing on well-being and stress (WHOQOL BREF questionnaire and Perceived Stress Scale (PSS)), and in-depth interviews	Pykett et al. [6]	2020a	Georeferenced data-involving people's personal opinions—the possibility of the participation of more people	The possibility of the influence of other conditions
14	Qualitative methods such as photovoice and pod walking	Versey [26]	2021	Involving people's personal opinions—the possibility of the participation of more people	The possibility of the influence of other conditions
15	Skin conductance response and visual stimuli from the environment	Garrett et al. [27]	2021	Georeferenced data	The small number of samples—the possibility of the influence of other conditions
16	Collaborative emotional maps which are created by showing emotions on them through emojis	Camara et al. [28]	2021	Involving people's personal opinions—the possibility of the participation of more people	The possibility of the influence of other conditions
17	Marking and specifying stressful points or calming points on analog maps	Adli et al. [29]	2016	Involving people's personal opinions—the possibility of the participation of more people	The possibility of the influence of other conditions

opinions, so, the use of methods such as biosensing in this field brings good advantages because the data used through this method can be very effectively georeferenced, making it possible to generate some maps showing the level of stress of citizens in each part of the city, if a sufficient number of samples are examined. However, there is also the possibility of the influence of other conditions in this method since issues like physical characteristics, other diseases, or individual conditions influence physiological signals. As another innovative method used in this field, one can refer to Android applications, that can be used by all citizens. Even, those, who suffer from urban stress, can use them to identify and choose the most relaxing route or the least stressful route. Moreover, the personal opinions of people with mental illness or stress are also very effective in this field, and it is necessary to consider them in the analysis of places in terms of urban stress.

According to the abovementioned, it is effective to use a combination of all these methods in the field of urban stress and their combination is the best option. The best urban stress measurement method is to combine the following methods: equipping places or subjects with devices such as biosensing, using applications with the capability of georeferencing data, using personal opinions of people, and interviewing people suffering from stress and mental illnesses.

References

1. Vojnovic I, Pearson A, Asiki G, Allen A, DeVerteuil G. Handbook of global urban health. 1st ed. Routledge; 2019. https://doi.org/10.4324/9781315465456.
2. Cappon D. Urban stress. CMA J. 1977;116:8.
3. Birenboim A, Dijst M, Scheepers FE, Poelman MP, Helbich M. Wearables and location tracking technologies for mental-state sensing in outdoor environments. Prof Geogr. 2019;71:449–61. https://doi.org/10.1080/00330124.2018.1547978.
4. Kyriakou K, Resch B. Spatial analysis of moments of stress derived from wearable sensor data. Adv Cartogr GIScience Int Cartogr Assoc. 2019;2:9. https://doi.org/10.5194/ica-adv-2-9-2019.
5. Zeile P, Resch B, Loidl M, Petutschnig A, Dörrzapf L. Urban emotions and cycling experience – enriching traffic planning for cyclists with human sensor data. GI Forum. 2016;1(1):204–16.
6. Pykett J, Osborne T, Resch B. From urban stress to neurourbanism: how should we research city well-being? Ann Am Assoc Geogr. 2020;2020:1–16. https://doi.org/10.1080/24694452.2020.1736982.
7. Bynion M, Feldner MT. Self-assessment manikin. Pers Individ Differ. 2017; https://doi.org/10.1007/978-3-319-28099-8_77-1.
8. Can YS, Arnrich B, Ersoy C. Stress detection in daily life scenarios using smart phones and wearable sensors: a survey. J Biomed Inform. 2019;92:103139. https://doi.org/10.1016/j.jbi.2019.103139.
9. McKay D. Computer-assisted and web-based innovations in psychology, special education, and health. Emerg Technol Clin Pract. 2016;2016:365–78. https://doi.org/10.1016/b978-0-12-802075-3.00014-0.
10. Gjoreski M, Luštrek M, Gams M, Gjoreski H. Monitoring stress with a wrist device using context. J Biomed Inform. 2017;73:159–70. https://doi.org/10.1016/j.jbi.2017.08.006.
11. Lee MY, Lee G, Bang S. Development stress monitoring system based on personal digital assistant (PDA). In: The 26th Annual International Conference of the IEEE Engineering in Medicine and Biology Society; 2004. p. 2364–7. https://doi.org/10.1109/IEMBS.2004.1403685.
12. Capineri C, Huang H, Gartner G. Tracking emotions in urban space. Two experiments in Vienna and Siena. Riv Geogr Ital. 2018;125(2):273–88.
13. Lin N, Lai G. Urban stress in China. Soc Sci Med. 1995;41(8):1131–45. https://doi.org/10.1016/0277-9536(94)00426-t.
14. Stockwell EG, Neal AG. A critique of the ZPG urban stress test: on the uses and misuses of social indicators. Soc Indic Res. 1991;24(4):393–402. https://doi.org/10.1007/bf00383736.

15. Kyriakou K, Resch B, Sagl G, Petutschnig A, Werner C, Niederseer D, et al. Detecting moments of stress from measurements of wearable physiological sensors. Sensors. 2019;19(17):3805. https://doi.org/10.3390/s19173805.
16. Baumann PS, Söderström O, Abrahamyan Empson L, Söderström D, Codeluppi Z, Golay P, et al. Urban remediation: a new recovery-oriented strategy to manage urban stress after first-episode psychosis. Soc Psychiatry Psychiatr Epidemiol. 2019;55:273–83. https://doi.org/10.1007/s00127-019-01795-7.
17. Reynolds LK, O'Koon JH, Papademetriou E, Szczygiel S, Grant KE. Stress and somatic complaints in low-income urban adolescents. J Youth Adolesc. 2001;30(4):499–514. https://doi.org/10.1023/a:1010401417828.
18. Nold C. Emotional cartography: technologies of the self. 2009. Emotional Cartography. Technologies of the Self (researchgate.net). Accessed 10 Sept 2021.
19. Bergner BS, Exner J-P, Memmel M, Raslan R, Talal M, Taha D, et al. Human sensory assessment linked with geo- and mobile-data processing methods in urban planning exemplified on different cultures in Germany and Egypt. In: Proceedings of CUPUM 2013: 13th International Conference on Computers in Urban Planning and Urban Management - Planning Support Systems for Sustainable Urban Development; 2013.
20. Huang H, Gartner G. Using mobile crowdsourcing and geotagged social media data to study people's affective responses to environments. In: Capineri C, Haklay M, Huang H, Antoniou V, Kettunen J, Ostermann F, Purves R, editors. European handbook of crowdsourced geographic information. London: Ubiquity Press; 2016. p. 383–97. https://doi.org/10.5334/bax.
21. Fathullah A, Willis K. Engaging the senses: the potential of emotional data for participation in urban planning. Urban Sci. 2018;2(4):98.
22. Chrisinger BW, King AC. Stress experiences in neighborhood and social environments (SENSE): a pilot study to integrate the quantified self with citizen science to improve the built environment and health. Int J Health Geogr. 2018;17(1):17. https://doi.org/10.1186/s12942-018-0140-1.
23. Werner C, Resch B, Loidl M. Evaluating urban bicycle infrastructures through intersubjectivity of stress sensations derived from physiological measurements. ISPRS Int J Geo Inf. 2019;8(6):265. https://doi.org/10.3390/ijgi8060265.
24. Neale C, Aspinall P, Roe J, Tilley S, Mavros P, Cinderby S, et al. The impact of walking in different urban environments on brain activity in older people. Cities Health. 2019;4:94–106. https://doi.org/10.1080/23748834.2019.1619893.
25. Teixeira IP, da Silva R, Schwanen T, Manzato GG, Dörrzapf L, Zeile P, et al. Does cycling infrastructure reduce stress biomarkers in commuting cyclists? A comparison of five European cities. J Transp Geogr. 2020;88:102830. https://doi.org/10.1016/j.jtrangeo.2020.102830.
26. Versey HS. Can mobile methods bridge psychology and place-based research? Qual Psychol. 2021;9:156–70. https://doi.org/10.1037/qup0000187.
27. Millar GC, Mitas O, Boode W, Hoeke L, de Kruijf J, Petrasova A, et al. Space-time analytics of human physiology for urban planning. Comput Environ Urban Syst. 2021;85:101554. https://doi.org/10.1016/j.compenvurbsys.2020.101554.
28. Camara GS, Camboim SP, Bravo JVM. Collaborative emotional mapping as a tool for urban mobility planning. Bull Geod Sci. 2021; https://doi.org/10.1590/s1982-21702021000s00011.
29. Adli M, Berger M, Brakemeier E-L, Engel L, Fingerhut J, Hehl R, et al. Neurourbanistik – ein methodischer Schulterschluss zwischen Stadtplanung und Neurowissenschaften. Die Psychiatrie. 2016;13:70–8.
30. Abrahamyan Empson L, Baumann PS, Söderström O, Codeluppi Z, Söderström D, Conus P. Urbanicity: the need for new avenues to explore the link between urban living and psychosis. Early Interv Psychiatry. 2019;14:398–409. https://doi.org/10.1111/eip.12861.
31. Knöll M, Neuheuser K, Cleff T, Rudolph-Cleff A. A tool to predict perceived urban stress in open public spaces. Environ Plan B Urban Anal City Sci. 2017;45:797–813. https://doi.org/10.1177/0265813516686971.

Chapter 6
Examining the Background and Global Experiences and Presenting Study Challenges and Gaps

Abstract This chapter consists of two sections: research background and global experiences. In the first section, the background of the research in urban mental health and urban stress is examined, and research challenges and gaps are presented. In the second section, global experiences related to urban mental health are explored, and issues and challenges are presented.

Since there is no global plan related to urban stress, this section provides some successful global experiences (Knox Mental Health Action Plan, Ararat City Municipal Public Health and Wellbeing Plan, Moreland municipal public health and wellbeing plan, Casey Municipal Public Health and Wellbeing Plan, Northern Grampians Municipal Public Health and Wellbeing Plan, Victorian Public Health and Wellbeing Plan) in the field of urban mental health improvement and the solutions presented in them are introduced. In fact, considering the relationship between the concepts of stress, health, mental health, and the city, cities reduce the mental health of citizens through urban stressors. So, the factors reducing urban mental health can be the same urban stressors. Of course, this issue needs further investigation. In the end, after examining global experiences, it has been tried to extract some stress-relief urban planning from these plans. In this section, it was attempted to examine the indicators presented in global experiences on the topic of urban mental health and collect the indicators corresponding to urban stress.

Keywords Environmental stress · Urban stress · Mental health

6.1 Introduction

This chapter consists of two sections: research background and global experiences. In the first section, the background of the research in urban mental health and urban stress is examined, and research challenges and gaps are presented. In the second section, global experiences related to urban mental health are explored, and issues and challenges are presented.

S. Jalilisadrabad et al., *Stress Relief Urban Planning*,
https://doi.org/10.1007/978-981-99-4202-2_6

6.2 Research Background

Issues such as mental health and stress are closely related. For this reason, this section examines the research background in two separate sections: urban mental health, and urban stress.

6.2.1 Background of Urban Mental Health

Since the research topic is urban stress, it has been attempted to introduce the most important studies in the field of urban mental health, with a significant influence on the research process, in Table 6.1.

Table 6.1 Research background in the field of urban mental health

	Research title	Authors	Year	Research purpose	Method	Results
1	*Mental disorders in urban areas: an ecological study of schizophrenia and other psychoses*	Faris and Dunham [1]	1939	To study mental disorders in patients in Chicago and the impact of urbanization on them	Exploratory	The relationship between urbanization and mental disorders was confirmed.
2	*Urban neighborhoods and mental health. Psychological contributions to understanding toxicity, resilience, and interventions*	Wandersman and Nation [2]	1998	To describe the relationship between structural characteristics of neighborhoods and mental health	Descriptive	This research discussed the effect of social, physical, and structural characteristics on different types of mental health outcomes, identified neighborhood characteristics reducing resilience, and investigated how psychology affects neighborhood interventions to improve neighborhood status.
3	*Housing and mental health: a review of the evidence and a methodological and conceptual critique*	Evans et al. [3]	2003	To identify methodological and conceptual shortcomings of theoretical literature on housing quality and mental health	Library	The findings include policy implications in this field of research.

Table 6.1 (continued)

	Research title	Authors	Year	Research purpose	Method	Results
4	*The current status of urban-rural differences in psychiatric disorders*	Peen et al. [4]	2010	To study urban-rural differences in psychiatric disorders	Meta-analysis	It was found that there is a significant pooled urban-rural odds ratio for the total prevalence of psychiatric disorders, and for mood disorders and anxiety disorders, and the prevalence of mental disorders was higher in the city.
5	*Neighborhood urban form, social environment, and depression*	Miles et al. [5]	2012	To study the relationship between the urban form of the neighborhood, and social environment, with depression symptoms	Exploratory	Living in neighborhoods with higher private car density, due to chronic noise, was associated with more stress symptoms.
6	*Cities and mental health*	Gruebner et al. [6]	2017	An overview of the risk factors of mental illness in urban centers	Library	Social isolation and social loneliness as well as poverty in the neighborhood contribute to the burden of mental health and more interdisciplinary research is needed to conclude.
7	*Urban social exclusion and mental health of China's rural-urban migrants—a review and call for research*	Li and Rose [7]	2017	To study the mental health of rural-urban migrants and its relationship with social exclusion	Descriptive-analytical	Social deprivation has reduced the mental health of migrants and limited access to full work rights, experience of social stigma, discrimination, and injustice are the most important factors.

(continued)

Table 6.1 (continued)

	Research title	Authors	Year	Research purpose	Method	Results
8	*Urban mental health*	Okkels et al. [8]	2018	To update urban mental health data and highlight challenges requiring immediate attention.	Library	Mental health challenges in urban areas include loneliness, violence, high crime rates, homelessness, noise and other pollutants, traffic accidents, drug abuse, and inadequate mental health services.
9	*Sociology, biology and mechanisms in urban mental health*	Manning [9]	2018	To examine the frequency of mental disorders in cities	Library	This research discussed seven examples of solutions and concluded that a more accurate ethnography is required to solve the problem.
10	*Urbanicity: the need for new avenues to explore the link between urban living and psychosis*	Abrahamyan Empson et al. [10]	2019	To survey, summarize and organize existing theoretical literature to identify research gaps for future studies	Library	New studies on urbanization should be more interdisciplinary (psychiatry, epidemiology, human geography, urban planning, etc.) to enrich research methods, develop treatment and preventive strategies appropriately, and also ensure the creation of urban environments that help people's mental well-being.
11	*Neighbourhood characteristics, prevalence, and severity of depression: pooled analysis of eight Dutch cohort studies*	Generaal et al. [11]	2019	To investigate the impact of urbanization, economic, physical, and social characteristics on the prevalence and intensity of depression	Descriptive-analytical	Urbanization and various economic, physical, and social characteristics of the neighborhood are associated with depression, indicating that a wide range of environmental aspects may be associated with poor mental health.

Table 6.1 (continued)

	Research title	Authors	Year	Research purpose	Method	Results
12	*Is urban living good for mental health?*	Lecic-Tosevski [12]	2019	To examine the mental health challenges of urban life and relevant perspectives	Library	The challenges of urban life are more in developing countries, and nature-based solutions may be useful in preventing mental disorders and the resulting psychological symptoms.
13	*Urbanization and emerging mental health issues*	Ventriglio et al. [13]	2020	A comprehensive review of emerging mental health issues related to urbanization and globalization processes	Library	Conducting further research and developing specific guidelines for improving mental health and mental health care facilities in cities are of great importance for policymakers and urban designers. Also, to prevent and reduce mental illnesses in cities, strategies should be adopted globally.
14	*Urbanicity mental costs valuation: a review and urban-societal planning consideration*	D'Acci et al. [14]	2020	To investigate the extent of economic savings in the world in case of improving urban mental health	Library	Better urban planning makes it possible to save about 1.2 trillion dollars yearly worldwide and even a reduction of only 20% in urban mental illness rate would save around 250 billion dollars yearly.
15	*Mental health in big cities*	Mari [15]	2020	To investigate the factors reducing mental health in big cities	Library	Future research should consider how these factors interact to make life better or worse for mental health in large cities.

(continued)

Table 6.1 (continued)

	Research title	Authors	Year	Research purpose	Method	Results
16	*Urbanization, urbanicity, and depression*	Sampson et al. [16]	2020	A systematic review of published studies on urbanization, urbanicity, and depression	Library	Urbanization may affect depression differently across geographic regions. The relationship between urbanization and depression is complicated and is likely mediated and moderated by many other factors.
17	*Urban sanity understanding urban mental health impacts and how to create saner*	Litman [17]	2021	To study how urban life affects the mental health and happiness of residents	Library	This report examined the specific mechanisms by which urban living can affect mental health and happiness and discussed the identity of practical strategies that can be used to increase urban mental health and happiness by communities and individuals.

Edward Shorter brought out the connection between living in an urban setting and mental problems in 1839. He discovered that metropolitan areas have a higher prevalence of mental diseases than suburban areas [8]. The findings of Faris and Dunham's seminal study on patients with mental problems admitted to psychiatric hospitals in Chicago between 1922 and 1934 were published in 1939. According to Faris and Dunham [1], they verified the link between urbanisation and mental problems. Faris and Dunham created the primary epidemiological work on mental illnesses and urban life. Additionally, they connected urban social problems with mental illnesses [9]. In the years that followed, numerous studies in the area of urban mental health were carried out using various methodologies. Seven strategies are revealed by a review of the literature on urban mental health: (1) exploratory studies that lead to the discovery of the relationship between urbanization and mental health, (2) library studies that attempt to summarize and organize theoretical foundations, (3) comparative studies that compare places, (4) detailed studies that address a specific problem or mental illness in cities, such as stress, depression, schizophrenia, etc., or the effects of mental health on a specific part of the city, such as housing, (5) studies that identify factors affecting urban mental health, (6) studies that provide specific guidelines influencing the subject, and (7) studies that are not included in the abovementioned six categories.

6.2.2 Background of Urban Stress

In this section, it was attempted to examine the background of urban stress. For this purpose, Table 6.2 presents the previous studies by the research title, authors, year, research purpose, method, and results.

Simmel's [18] seminal thesis served as the foundation for the study of urban stress. In the late nineteenth century, he hypothesised variables including sensitivity to noise and air pollution and saw the modern metropolis as an ineluctable psychologically stimulating environment. Simmel attempted to create two fields of study: the study of urban effects (as the study of psychological stimulation and the measurement of its effects) and the study of urban rhythms (as the study of individual brain stimulation) [18]. In the 1950s and 1960s, while Simmel's ideas were developing, Prindle recognized urban stress as the current disease of cities and considered it a disease caused by overcrowding, the most effective solution of which is to identify possible sources [19]. Next, Milgram [20] proposed the perspective of stimulus overload and adaptation strategies, analogized the city to the frozen world, and introduced the concept of familiar strangers [20]. Christmas [22] discussed the necessity of developing health services according to environmental stress [22]. Then, Lazarus and Cohen [23] emphasized the importance of studying environmental stress in real conditions and considered the laboratory inappropriate for this research [23]. Also, Burton [27] emphasized the necessity of longitudinal studies in this field [27]. Considering the approved relationship between urbanization and mental health by Faris and Dunham and the approved relationship between urbanization and stress by Simmel, this effect was proven by Lederbogen et al. [35] in a laboratory ambiance using brain imaging [35]. In 2016, the term "neuro urbanism" was proposed for the first time as a solution to urban stress, which resulted in the "Charta of Neurourbanism" in 2019 [43].

Since the beginning of the twentieth century, many studies have investigated the relationship between urbanization and stress and provided effective solutions to it with different approaches. However, no study has been carried out to develop stress-relief urban planning so far. Most studies have examined only part of the subject and have provided effective solutions in the same subject.

Table 6.2 Research background in the field of urban stress

	Research title	Author(s)	Year	Research purpose	Method	Results
1	*The metropolis and mental life*	Simmel [18]	1903	To examine the relationship between mental health and the environment	Descriptive-analytical	The study of urban stress for the first time and the analysis of urban effects (as the science of psychological stimulation and the measurement of its effects) and the analysis of urban rhythms (as the science of individual brain stimulation) are among the findings of this research.
2	*Health aspects of the urban environment*	Prindle [19]	1968	To study the health aspects of the environment	Library	Urban stress was recognized as the current disease of cities and introduced as a disease caused by overcrowding, the most effective solution of which is to identify possible sources.
3	*The experience of living in cities*	Milgram [20]	1970	To describe and analyze New York City	Descriptive-analytical	The perspective of stimulus overload and adaptation strategies were raised, the city was analogized to the frozen world, and the concept of familiar strangers was introduced.
4	*Urban stress. experiments on noise and social stressors*	Proshansky [21]	1972	To examine the effects of stressors such as noise	Exploratory	This research examined the self-control power of people in different stressful situations and introduced social interference as a factor to reduce the self-control power of a person.
5	*Psychological stresses of urban living: new direction for mental health services in the inner city*	Christmas [22]	1973	To clarify the need for a comprehensive operational framework for mental health promotion	Descriptive	Health services should be developed to help social units to deal with environmental stress and the physical, social, economic, and psychological behavior of urbanites must be considered.

6	*Environmental stress*	Lazarus and Cohen [23]	1977	To study stress as part of the complicated relationship between the individual and the environment	Library	To reach a more accurate conclusion, it is required to study people in daily life conditions, many times intensively, to get a valid credit. Emphasis on the deep picture of social, psychological, and physiological processes and sustainable patterns in the real world instead of the laboratory.
7	*Rural-urban differences in the use of stress-alleviative drugs*	Webb and Collette [24]	1977	To investigate the use of stress-alleviative drugs as a marker of stress in rural and urban areas	Descriptive-analytical	Stress-related disorders are much more common among rural than urban dwellers.
8	*Stress and the environment*	Baum et al. [25]	1981	Overview of the literature on stress and the environment	Library	Despite its general usage, stress refers to a process that is not only specific but central to the relationship between people and their surroundings.
9	*Environmental stress and cognitive performance*	Cohen et al. [26]	1986	Overview of environmental stress	Library	Environmental stress and its relationship with human behavior and health were addressed.
10	*Factors in urban stress*	Burton [27]	1990	To investigate changes in health patterns, causes and effects of urban stress, and stress management approaches	Explanatory	Detailed planning and longitudinal comparisons are needed to obtain the necessary feedback for policy evaluation and modification.
11	*Urban stress in China*	Lin and Lai [28]	1995	To examine the stress model in an urban center named Tianjin	Descriptive-analytical	Both the generality of the stress-distress model and the specificity of the effects of work-related stressors were supported.

(continued)

Table 6.2 (continued)

	Research title	Author(s)	Year	Research purpose	Method	Results
12	*Chronic aircraft noise exposure, stress responses, mental health and cognitive performance in school children*	Haines et al. [29]	2001	To study the effects of aircraft noise exposure on children around London Heathrow Airport in terms of stress responses, mental health, and cognitive performance	Descriptive-analytical	Chronic aircraft noise exposure is associated with impaired comprehension and high noise levels but not mental health problems in children, and factors such as social class and deprivation play a mediating role here.
13	*Race, urban community stressors, and behavioral and emotional problems of children with special health care needs*	Jaffee et al. [30]	2005	To investigate the relationship between urban stressors and behavioral and emotional problems of African-American and white children in need of health care	Descriptive-analytical (interview)	Primary care providers may be better able to identify important exacerbating factors with an urban stress assessment. In this context, auxiliary care systems are needed in dealing with stressors at the level of urban society.
14	*Correlates of urban stress and mental health: the impact of social context on resilience*	Miller and Phillips [31]	2005	To investigate how to promote individual resilience to protect against chronic stress vulnerability	Library	The relationship between lack of basic support, lack of opportunity structures, and mental health problems, is not linear, but a process involving stress and emotional social deprivation. Thus, financial resources alone cannot prevent high levels of mental illness.
15	*Urban stress and health in developing countries: development and validation of a neighborhood stress index for India*	Suchday et al. [32]	2006	To assess stress as a function of environmental conditions	Descriptive-analytical (confirmatory factor analysis)	This study provides preliminary evidence of the relationship between stress and health that should be further explored. It is critical to identify lifestyle-related disorders in India's growing population and behavioral and psychosocial factors that can be modified and may form the basis of prevention programs.

16	*Stress and the city: housing stressors are associated with respiratory health among low socioeconomic status Chicago children*	Quinn et al. [33]	2010	To evaluate the impact of urban stress on the aggravation of asthma symptoms	Descriptive Analytical Exploratory	The results contributed to the conceptualization of urban stress as a "social pollutant" and the hypothetical role of stress in health differences. The findings provided interventions to improve asthma outcomes and structural solutions for residential stressors and health inequities.
17	*Urban stress and mental health*	Adli [34]	2011	To briefly describe the relationship between stress, mental health, and urbanization	Library	This challenge, which is known as the twenty-first-century challenge, can be solved by joint action between life sciences, social sciences, urban planning, architecture, and politics.
18	*City living and urban upbringing affect neural social stress processing in humans*	Lederbogen et al. [35]	2011	Laboratory evaluation of the effects of urbanization on the human brain	Experimental	Cities negatively influence mental health, and mood and anxiety disorders are more common in cities, and schizophrenia has greatly increased in people who were born or lived in cities.
19	*The concrete jungle: city stress and substance abuse among young adult African American men*	Seth et al. [36]	2012	To investigate the relationship between urban stress, alcohol consumption, and drug use among African-American men	Exploratory	African American men living within a stressful urban environment are at increased risk of exposure to and use of illicit substances. Culturally competent public health interventions to control drug use should address psychological factors such as stress and neighborhood violence.

(continued)

Table 6.2 (continued)

	Research title	Author(s)	Year	Research purpose	Method	Results
20	*Urban environmental stress and behavioral adaptation in Bhopal City of India*	Rishi and Khuntia [37]	2012	To investigate perceived urban environmental stressors and coping strategies adopted by people to cope with the results of urban environmental stress	Explanatory	The results indicated that city planners should reduce the effect of stressors using various interventions. This paper provided guidelines for other cities to develop environmental competence and generate collective awareness about urban environmental stress and its possible management options to help people develop environmental resilience and functional coping.
21	*Urban social stress—risk factor for mental disorders*	Lederbogen et al. [38]	2013	To understand social stress as a risk factor for mental disorders among citizens	Multivariate analysis	To understand how social stress acts as a risk factor for mental disorders in citizens, factors such as social status, environmental pollutants, infrastructure, and economic issues should be considered.
22	*Stress and the city*	Steinheuser et al. [39]	2014	To investigate the relationship between urban upbringing and the activity of the hypothalamus-pituitary-adrenal (HPA) axis, which is one of the stress response systems	Descriptive	According to the findings, urban upbringing is associated with increased cortisol response to acute stress.
23	*Einflussfaktoren der gebauten Umwelt auf wahrgenommene Aufenthaltsqualität bei der Nutzung städtischer Räume*	Knöll et al. [40]	2014	To identify problematic spaces and to categorize relevant urban aspects	Descriptive-analytical	This research provided a basis for identifying problematic and stressful spaces with special characteristics. In further studies, psychophysiological measurements can be used to objectively evaluate such factors.

24	*The stress of the street for patients with persecutory delusions: a test of the symptomatic and psychological effects of going outside into a busy urban area*	Freeman et al. [41]	2015	To examine the symptomatic and psychological effects of going outside into a busy urban area	Descriptive-analytical	Compared with staying inside, the street exposure condition resulted in significant increases in paranoia, voices, anxiety, negative beliefs about the self, and negative beliefs about others. This exposure also resulted in a decrease in positive thoughts about the self.
25	*Stress in the city: influence of urban social stress and violence on pregnancy and postpartum quality of life among adolescent and young mothers*	Willie et al. [42]	2016	To study the impact of the urban social environment (stressful incidents, discrimination, and neighborhood problems) on the quality of life of mothers	Descriptive-analytical	The results of the structural equation and multi-group models showed that higher urban social stress predicts lower mental and physical quality of life during pregnancy and after pregnancy and there is a need to stress reduction programs to help young mothers in urban areas.
26	*Neurourbanistik – ein methodischer Schulterschluss zwischen Stadtplanung und Neurowissenschaften*	Adli et al. [43]	2016	To introduce Neurourbanism and its study challenges	Library	An interdisciplinary approach between architecture, urban planning, neuroscience, and medicine was introduced under the proposed term "neuro-urbanism".
28	*Revealed: the world's least stressful cities*	Knöll et al. [44]	2017	To predict perceived urban stress ratings in Darmstadt, Germany	Exploratory Multivariate analysis	The types of public open space (park, square, yard, street), isovist characteristics, street network characteristics, and building density are the most important predictors for perceived urban stress, respectively.

(continued)

Table 6.2 (continued)

	Research title	Author(s)	Year	Research purpose	Method	Results
29	*A tool to predict perceived urban stress in open public spaces*	Mubi Brighenti and Pavoni [45]	2017	To describe the complicated issue of urban stress (a brief description of the history of urban stress from Simmel to 2016)	Library	Adaptation strategies to stressful environments are not simply a matter of personal taste or individual choices. To understand an ecological approach, paying attention to the urban-ecological combination should complement a phenomenological approach to the intersubjective experience.
30	*City of unpleasant feelings. Stress, comfort and animosity in urban life*	Söderström et al. [46]	2017	To investigate how to manage the problems created by the urban environment for people	Descriptive-analytical	Systematic analysis of interviews and observations shows that the tactics are categorized into three groups: programming and regulating mobility, creating a bubble of isolation, and creating an atmosphere of comfort.
31	*Emplacing recovery: how persons diagnosed with psychosis handle stress in cities, psychosis*	Elsamahy and Abd El-Fattah [47]	2018	To evaluate public spaces in terms of users' activity concerning stressors, in the city of Tripoli, Lebanon	Analytical	Development of a methodology for designing stress-free public spaces.
32	*Designing non-stressed psychological public spaces*	Mukherjee and Agrawal [48]	2018	To study the influence of urban stress factors on ground cover vegetation	Descriptive-analytical	Three characteristics of air pollution, land use type, and soil properties showed significant variability among sites in terms of vegetation.

33	*The influence of urban stress factors on responses of ground cover vegetation*	Li and Liu [49]	2018	To investigate the mental health impact of housing disadvantages concerning the migrant population in China, who are largely excluded from the formal housing sector.	Descriptive-analytical (survey)	Poor housing conditions are significantly associated with perceived stress but not with mental health, while the neighborhood social environment significantly predicts both perceived stress and mental health. Also, there is a need for more ethnographic research on migrant resilience and stress-coping strategies to address mental health in migrant settlements.
34	*Housing stress and mental health of migrant populations in urban China*	Chrisinger and King [50]	2018	To identify visible and invisible environmental elements causing chronic stress in the urban environment using the combination of biosensing data and citizen science	Descriptive-analytical	This review paves the way for further research on combining qualitative and quantitative data on the built environment and urban stress. It also provides a systematic process for the simultaneous collection of multiple types of data and offers a basis for future spatial and statistical analyses, in addition to a deeper interpretation of how these responses differ within and between individuals.
35	*Stress experiences in neighborhood and social environments (SENSE): a pilot study to integrate the quantified self with citizen science to improve the built environment and health*	Baumann et al. [10]	2019	To study a set of possible strategies to help promote mental health and reduce urban stress	Descriptive-analytical	These possible strategies to help promote mental health and reduce urban stress in cities were categorized under the term "urban remediation" and how they affect patients to improve mental health was discussed.

(continued)

Table 6.2 (continued)

	Research title	Author(s)	Year	Research purpose	Method	Results
36	*Urban remediation: a new recovery-oriented strategy to manage urban stress after first-episode psychosis*	Fett et al. [51]	2019	To review studies in the fields of mental health and urban stress	Library	The mechanisms underlying the effects of urbanization on psychosis risk remain largely unknown and should be explored in global, multidisciplinary (neuro urbanism) research efforts.
37	*Psychosis and urbanicity*	Kyriakou and Resch [52]	2019	To propose a method for spatial analysis of moments of stress (MOS)	Descriptive-analytical	After conducting two field studies in the real world, it was found that the proposed approach can identify spatial patterns according to stress in urban areas.
38	*Spatial analysis of moments of stress derived from wearable sensor data*	Meloni et al. [53]	2019	To study the role of urban stress, local identity, and sustainability worldviews in predicting a set of pro-environmental behaviors in the urban context	Exploratory	The results show that both urban stress and endorsement of sustainability worldviews are significant positive predictors of pro-environmental behavior. City identity moderates the relationship between urban stress and the tendency to pay for green energy and lack of waste generation, respectively.
39	*Predicting pro-environmental behaviors in the urban context: The direct or moderated effect of urban stress, city identity, and worldviews*	Werner et al. [54]	2019	To investigate the feeling of stress through the quantification of physiological measurements	Descriptive-analytical	The findings are related to supporting more informed decision-making in urban planning with new data-driven applications in the field of smart cities to find sustainable solutions for various urban issues.

40	*Evaluating urban bicycle infrastructures through intersubjectivity of stress sensations derived from physiological measurements*	Birenboim et al. [55]	2019	To investigate the theoretical and practical aspects of using ambulatory devices to detect the mental state of people in open spaces with an emphasis on stress	Descriptive	Despite the challenges and limitations of current sensors, the use of these devices offers novel opportunities to assess physiological signals as markers of psychological state and stress. This research examines the performance of combining the sensor (Empatica E4) with GPS to measure stress.
41	*Wearables and location tracking technologies for mental-state sensing in outdoor environments*	Pykett et al. [56]	2020	To study emerging conceptual and methodological discussions of urban stress	Library	Biosensing data can be used to clarify narrative data related to social and political aspects.
42	*From urban stress to neurourbanism: how should we research city well-being?*	Pykett et al. [57]	2020	To investigate the potential and future challenges for developing an interdisciplinary and mixed citizen social science approach with an emphasis on urban stress for research on urban emotions	Library	Novel methods, such as biosensors for researching urban stress, face several ethical, political, and conceptual challenges. Also, issues such as strictness, participation, and social scientific interpretation are among their problems. Citizen social science methods can create more effective ways to address urban stress and promote well-being in urban communities.
43	*Developing a citizen social science approach to understand urban stress and promote wellbeing in urban communities*	Adli and Schondorf [58]	2020	To introduce a method to study stress in cities	Library	To study stress, an interdisciplinary research approach combining urban research, medicine, and neuroscience and promoting knowledge exchange with politics, civil society, and citizens in a transdisciplinary manner must be adopted.

(continued)

Table 6.2 (continued)

	Research title	Author(s)	Year	Research purpose	Method	Results
44	*Does the city make us ill? The effect of urban stress on emotions, behavior, and mental health*	Vargas et al. [59]	2020	To investigate types of structural exposure to stress	Library	The findings indicated three types of structural exposure to stress (stimulation by urban environments and their characteristics, exposure to differences, and exposure to environments lacking economic and social resources). Determining the cause of stress at the level of systems is effective in reducing barriers to effective interventions and health policy.
45	*Chronic stress, structural exposures and neurobiological mechanisms: a stimulation, discrepancy and deprivation model of psychosis*	Shannon et al. [60]	2020	To investigate the relationship between neighborhood crime and violence and stress in pregnant women	Descriptive-analytical	Regardless of race, neighborhood violent crime is associated with high levels of perceived stress in an urban cohort and pregnant women.
46	*Neighborhood violent crime and perceived stress in pregnancy*	Hernandez et al. [61]	2020	To simultaneously examine intrapersonal characteristics (distress tolerance) and interpersonal characteristics (social support) and their relationships with urban stress	Descriptive-analytical	Findings suggested that interventions aimed at increasing social support may also increase distress tolerance skills and indirectly reduce depression symptoms in the context of urban stress among adults experiencing homelessness.
47	*Urban stress indirectly influences psychological symptoms through its association with distress tolerance and perceived social support among adults experiencing homelessness*	Evans et al. [62]	2020	To investigate the relationship between urbanicity and mental health problems directly and indirectly through the biological stress system functioning	Descriptive-analytical	The findings provided evidence of the relationship between urbanicity, biological stress system functioning, and mental health problems. To investigate environmental effects, long-term biological stress levels should be measured.

48	*Urbanicity, biological stress system functioning and mental health in adolescents*	Dykas et al. [63]	2021	To examine the relationship between urban stress and early adolescents behavior	Descriptive-analytical	After controlling for demographic factors, it was found that there is a positive relationship between early adolescents' risk-taking propensity and affiliation with risky peers and high levels of urban stress but not with low levels of urban stress.
49	*Early adolescents' risk taking propensity, urban stress, and affiliation with risky peers*	Buttazzoni et al. [64]	2021	To examine the relationship between public health, planning, and neuro urbanism	Analytical	Proposing two new conceptual frameworks (research-oriented and practice-oriented), which focus on the relationship between urban environments and the mental health of the youth and can help direct practices and future research in this field.

6.3 Global Experiences

Considering the connections between the concepts of stress, health, and mental health, cities reduce citizens' mental health through urban stressors because there is no global strategy to address urban stress. This section provides some successful global experiences in the area of improving urban mental health, and the solutions presented in them are introduced. So, the factors reducing urban mental health can be the same as urban stars'lessorss. Of course, this issue needs further investigation. In the end, after examining global experiences, it has been tried to extract some stress-relief urban planning from these plans.

6.3.1 The Knox Mental Health Action Plan (2021–2025)

6.3.1.1 Introduction of the Plan

The Knox Mental Health Action Plan (2021–2025) was developed and approved in 2021 for 4 years by the Knox city council. It was designed to give the Knox community a strategic framework for addressing present and future mental health issues, facilitate community intervention coordination, and address both continuing city needs and the effects of COVID-19 [65]. In comparison to the Victorian average, Knox inhabitants reported higher rates of psychological distress as well as poorer levels of life satisfaction in 2017. Additionally, almost 25% of Knox City citizens have experienced anxiety or depression at some point in their lives [65]. Investigations carried out in 2020 revealed that Knox City citizens' mental health had significantly declined over the previous 4 years, and problems like the HIV/AIDS pandemic had made matters worse. The Knox City Council has made the decision to take a more aggressive stance in its strategy for this reason [65]. This idea is briefly introduced in Fig. 6.1.

The Knox mental health action plan

Origin of plan: State of Victoria, Australia

City Population: 163203 people **City Area:** 114 km^2

Period: 2021-2025

Administered by: Knox City Council

Approved by: Knox City Council and Community Wellbeing Department

Plan purpose: to provide a strategic framework to address the current and emerging mental health needs of the Knox community, help coordinate interventions in the community, and respond to the consequences of Knox 19 and the ongoing needs of the city [67].

Fig. 6.1 Introduction of The Knox mental health action plan

6.3.1.2 Actions and Policies of the Plan

This strategy focuses on three levels of prevention: primary prevention (preventing the onset of a condition by preventing it from happening in the first place), secondary prevention (focusing on diagnosing and treating a mental health condition at its earliest stage to reduce its duration and severity), and tertiary prevention (reducing the impact of an established risk on a person's functioning, quality of life, and longevity through treatment and psychosocial support). In fact, this plan seeks to identify the interventions that should be made after the introduction of protective factors and risk factors in order to lessen the risk factors and increase the protective factors because the urban dweller will experience psychological issues if the balance of these factors is upset [65]. The interventions are:

Structural
- Safe and secure living environment
- Equality and tolerance
- Access to support services

Social and economic
- Positive early attachment
- Responsive parenting, monitoring and involvement
- Personal safety
- Social support and confiding relationships
- Positive community recovery and resilience following disasters such as natural disasters and drought

Individual
- Educational outcomes
- Self confidence
- Problem solving and communication skills
- Ability to handle stress
- Good physical health

6.3.2 Ararat City Municipal Public Health and Wellbeing Plan (2013–2017)

6.3.2.1 Introduction of the Plan

The Ararat City Council's strategic plan to advance community health is the Ararat City Municipal Public Health and Wellbeing Plan 2013–2017 [66]. One of the best healthcare systems in the world is found in Australia. The Public Health and Welfare Act of 2008 mandates that councils work to safeguard, enhance, and promote the public's health and wellbeing within their municipal catchment. Following the passing of this law, Victoria's cities created Municipal Public Health and Well-being

Ararat City Municipal Public Health and Wellbeing Plan

Origin of plan: State of Victoria, Australia

City Population: 11795 people **City Area:** 4211 km^2

Period: 2013-2017

Administered by: Ararat City Council

Plan purpose: to describe how the Ararat Rural City Council will work to improve the health and well-being of the local community over the next four years [68].

Fig. 6.2 Introduction of public health and welfare plan of Ararat City Municipal Public Health and Wellbeing Plan

Plans (MPHWPs), which include a section on mental health [66]. This strategy is simply explained in Fig. 6.2.

6.3.2.2 Actions and Policies of the Plan

This plan includes the built environment (urban planning features, housing, parks, roads, and transport modes that foster access, belonging, and social inclusion), economic (employment, economic policy, e.g. rural reduction), natural (the presence of natural vegetation for promoting recreation, leisure, and contact with nature), and social (the cost of community building initiatives, community facilities, and support programs, artistic and cultural programs) factors affecting mental health [66] and addresses some issues such as increasing healthy nutrition, increasing physical activity, controlling tobacco use, improving oral health, reducing alcohol and drug abuse, promoting sexual and reproductive health, promoting mental health, preventing damage, and preventing skin cancer [66]. In the mental health section of this plan, the improvement of mental health is addressed through increasing social relations and the actions of the council are introduced as follows:

1. To create opportunities to promote community pride, a sense of belonging, and participation.
2. To provide support for community development and collaborative projects.
3. To support social diversity and cultural events.
4. To pursue initiatives promoting lifelong learning, literacy, and information needs of society.
5. To support and develop youth development programs and services.

6. To support the police and community safety programs and relevant initiatives.
7. To promote Ararat Performing Arts Center and its diverse performing arts program.
8. To develop the Ararat regional art gallery.
9. To provide a diverse and accessible innovative program of related exhibitions and events within the performing and visual arts programs.
10. To use and develop lands to support social, economic, and environmental well-being.
11. To maintain facilities in favor of the whole community.
12. To support mental health and well-being initiatives in early childhood settings, schools, and workplaces through the Healthy Together Achievement Program [66].

6.3.3 *Moreland Municipal Public Health and Wellbeing Plan (2017–2021)*

6.3.3.1 Introduction of the Plan

The Moreland municipal public health and wellbeing plan 2017–2021 was developed and approved in 2021 by the Moreland City Council. It aimed to improve the health, livability, and sustainability of Moreland City [67]. Since this plan aimed to promote health, only part of it addressed the issue of mental health. Figure 6.3 briefly introduces this plan.

Moreland municipal public health and wellbeing plan

Origin of plan: Melbourne, Australia

City population: 181,725 people, **City Area:** 51 km^2

Period: 2017-2021

Administered by: Moreland City Council

Plan purpose: to promote health (high physical activity, healthy food, healthy society, safety, low drug use, available learning opportunities, and high mental health), livability (access to daily needs on foot, growing economy growth, diverse housing, adequate facilities and public space, high access to open space, encouraging social. interaction, and integrated transportation) and sustainability

Fig. 6.3 Introduction of Moreland municipal public health and wellbeing plan

6.3.3.2 Actions and Policies of the Plan

This plan has taken steps to improve mental health by focusing on the following 4-year priorities.

1. To strengthen the organizational understanding of the concepts of mental health and well-being, as the factors protecting people against mental illness, and to understand how social determinants can affect mental health.
2. To support the mental health and well-being of residents through regional partnerships and social determinants of health at the community level.
3. To enhance citizens' understanding of the factors affecting their mental health and well-being and to improve access to the services they need.
4. To cooperate with organizations, in projects and campaigns promoting the mental health and well-being of residents.
5. To measure the mental health of residents and to support those who participate in projects [67].

6.3.4 Casey Municipal Public Health and Wellbeing Plan (2017–2021)

6.3.4.1 Introduction of the Plan

The Casey Municipal Public Health and Wellbeing Plan 2017–2021 was developed in 2017 by the Casey City Council, the Department of Health, Treatment, and Human Services in the South, and the Women's Health Organization in the South East [68]. Casey is one of the cities of the state of Victoria, Australia, which is located in the suburbs of Melbourne. This plan, like the previous two plans, was prepared based on the Public Health and Welfare Act 2008. Figure 6.4 introduces this plan.

Casey Municipal Public Health and Wellbeing Plan

Origin of Plan: Melbourne, Australia

City Population: 340,419 people, **City Area:** 409 km^2

Period: 2017-2021

Administered by: Casey City Council, the Department of Health, Treatment, and Human Services in the South, and Women's Health Organization in the South East

Plan purpose: to protect and support the health and well-being of the Casey community by focusing on preventable risk factors affecting chronic health conditions [70].

Fig. 6.4 Introduction of Casey municipal public health and wellbeing plan

6.3.4.2 Actions and Policies of the Plan

Improving mental health is one of the overall goals of this strategy, which includes goals like boosting social inclusion and community resilience, raising participation levels in society, and supporting a calculated strategy to tackle the issue. Electronic gaming machines, diversity policy, access and inclusion, Casey's comprehensive strategic framework, the policy of access to community facilities, a community interaction strategy, a community resilience plan, a voluntary participation strategy, an art development plan, a child, youth, and family plan, and a native engagement plan were just a few of the strategies that were put forth to accomplish these goals [68].

6.3.5 Northern Grampians Municipal Public Health and Wellbeing Plan (2017–2021)

6.3.5.1 Introduction of the Plan

The Northern Grampians Municipal Public Health and Wellbeing Plan 2017–2021 was developed in 2017 by the Northern Grampians city council [69]. Figure 6.5 briefly introduces this plan.

6.3.5.2 Actions and Policies of the Plan

Since improving mental and subjective well-being is one of the goals of the plan, the following strategies have been proposed to achieve this goal.

1. To reduce the stigma of diseases related to mental health.
2. To develop resilience in all stages of society's life.

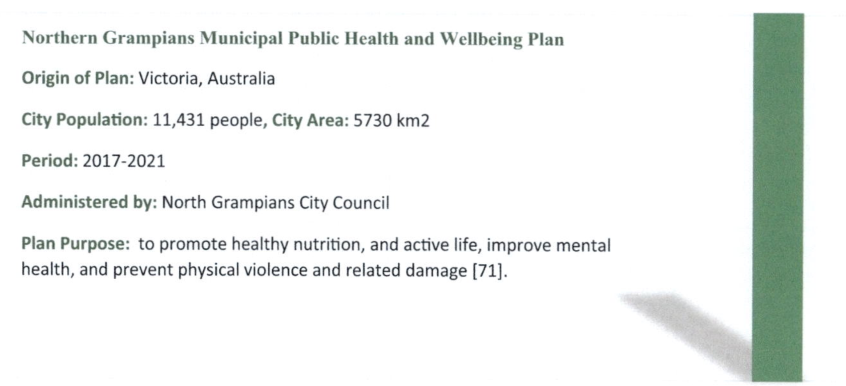

Fig. 6.5 Introduction of the Northern Grampians municipal public health and wellbeing plan

3. To promote services and access to them for people who need support by improving mental health.
4. To support the community to develop an empowerment strategy in social tenure, health, and well-being opportunities.
5. To encourage interaction in natural environments [69].

6.3.6 *Victorian Public Health and Well-Being Plan*

6.3.6.1 Introduction of the Plan

The Victorian Public Health and Wellbeing Plan was developed for the state of Victoria in three 4-year periods (2011–2015), (2015–2019), and (2019–2023). This plan is one of the macro plans at the state level, but its mental health part plays a significant role in the development of this research. Figure 6.6 introduces this plan.

6.3.6.2 Actions and Policies of the Plan

In its mental health section, this plan has stated the following policies and strategies in each period to improve mental health in the state.

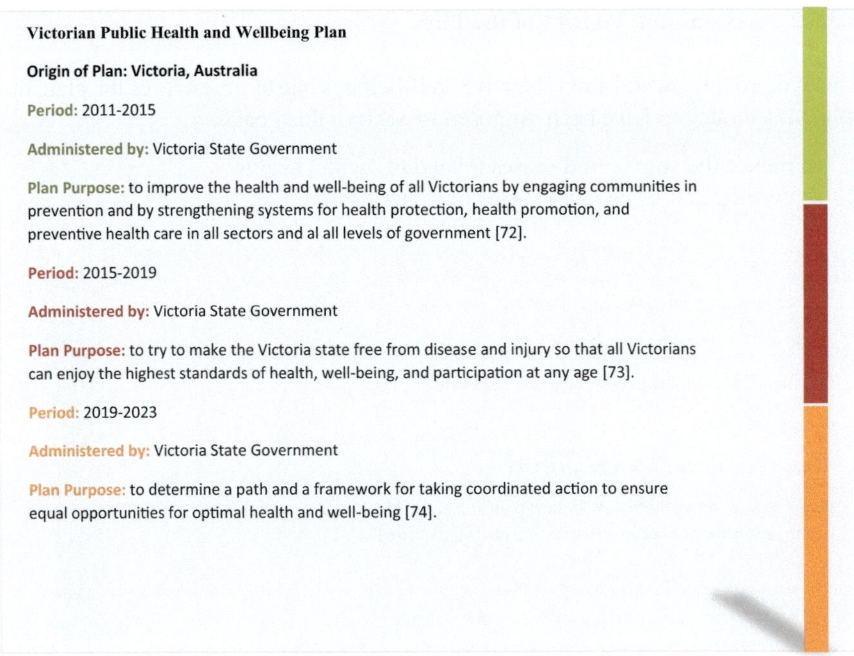

Fig. 6.6 Introduction of the Victorian public health and well-being plan

Actions (2011–2015):

1. Through a collaborative approach to mental health promotion (including stress management at work, preventing violence against women, and encouraging acceptance of diversity and social inclusion to build resilient and connected communities), protective factors for mental health will be strengthened and risk factors will be decreased.
2. To target mental illnesses and suicide prevention measures.
3. To develop resources to support mental health enhancement in local communities, workplaces, and early childhood services and schools.
4. To try to improve resilience.
5. To develop suicide prevention strategies [70].

Actions (2015–2019):

1. To improve and develop approaches like addressing discrimination, promoting contact with the natural environment, encouraging positive body image, lowering disordered eating, preventing violence against women, managing workplace stress, raising participation in physical activity and sports, and promoting acceptance of diversity and social inclusion in order to create resilient and connected communities.
2. To increase the intensity of targeted action for people with social and economic weaknesses.
3. To invest in early identification and intervention for vulnerable children and families.
4. To focus on the promotion of well-being and the prevention of suicide [71].

Actions (2019–2023):

1. To reduce the prevalence of mental illnesses, and to increase resilience among individuals, families, and communities.
2. To reduce the social gap and increase social communication.
3. To try to reduce the suicide rate [72].

6.3.7 Summary of Global Experiences

In this section, it was attempted to examine the indicators presented in global experiences on the topic of urban mental health and collect the indicators corresponding to urban stress, as presented in Table 6.3. After examining the global successful experiences, indicators of improving residents' self-confidence, suicide rate, community resilience, familiarity with coping skills, and the status of cultural and artistic events were identified as new, unexpressed indicators of urban stressors.

Table 6.3 Summary of global experiences

Effective indicators	Knox mental health action plan	Ararat city municipal public health and wellbeing plan	Moreland municipal public health and wellbeing plan	Casey municipal public health and wellbeing plan	Northern Grampians municipal public health and wellbeing plan	Victorian public health and wellbeing plan	Frequency
Access to mental health support services	*		*	*	*		4
Equality and civility	*						1
Creating a safe and secure living environment	*	*					2
Positively improving community and resilience following disasters such as natural disasters and droughts	*			*	*	*	4
Promoting social support and inclusion	*			*		*	4
Reducing social discrimination						*	1
Problem-solving and improving communication skills	*						1
Improving the ability to deal with stress and coping skills	*		*				2
Improving residents' self-confidence	*					*	
Reducing drug use	*						1
Reducing poverty and economic insecurity	*						1

Table 6.3 (continued)

Effective indicators	Knox mental health action plan	Ararat city municipal public health and wellbeing plan	Moreland municipal public health and wellbeing plan	Casey municipal public health and wellbeing plan	Northern Grampians municipal public health and wellbeing plan	Victorian public health and wellbeing plan	Frequency
Resolving issues concerning immigration and resettlement	*						1
Reducing exposure to violence	*						1
Creating opportunities to promote community pride, a sense of belonging, and participation		*	*	*		*	4
Providing support for community development and collaborative projects		*				*	2
Supporting cultural and art events		*		*			2
Pursuing initiatives that promote literacy and information needs of society and educating and empowering different groups of society	*	*					3
Supporting and developing youth programs and services		*					1

(continued)

Table 6.3 (continued)

Effective indicators	Knox mental health action plan	Ararat city municipal public health and wellbeing plan	Moreland municipal public health and wellbeing plan	Casey municipal public health and wellbeing plan	Northern Grampians municipal public health and wellbeing plan	Victorian public health and wellbeing plan	Frequency
Using and developing lands to support social, economic, and environmental well-being		*					1
Supporting mental health and well-being initiatives in early childhood settings, schools, and workplaces through the Healthy Together Achievement Program		*		*		*	3
Measuring the mental well-being of residents and supporting those who participate in projects			*				1
Promoting diversity in urban environments		*		*		*	3
Reducing the stigma of diseases related to mental health					*		1
Encouraging interaction with natural environments					*	*	2

Table 6.3 (continued)

Effective indicators	Knox mental health action plan	Ararat city municipal public health and wellbeing plan	Moreland municipal public health and wellbeing plan	Casey municipal public health and wellbeing plan	Northern Grampians municipal public health and wellbeing plan	Victorian public health and wellbeing plan	Frequency
Supporting the community to develop an empowerment strategy in social tenure, health, and well-being opportunities					*		1
Developing suicide prevention strategies						*	1
Increasing the intensity of targeted action for people with social and economic weaknesses						*	1
Promoting physical activities						*	1

6.4 Conclusion

Since the beginning of the twentieth century, many studies have investigated the relationship between urbanization and stress and provided effective solutions to it with different approaches. However, no study has been carried out to develop stress-relief urban planning so far. Most studies have examined only part of the subject and have provided effective solutions in the same subject. The review of global experiences also shows that no stress-relief urban plan or no urban design has been carried out. One of the reasons for this issue is the insufficient theoretical foundations in this field. After examining the global successful experiences, indicators of improving residents' self-confidence, suicide rate, community resilience, familiarity with coping skills, and the status of cultural and artistic events were identified as new, unexpressed indicators of urban stressors.

References

1. Faris REL, Dunham HW. Mental disorders in urban areas: an ecological study of schizophrenia and other psychoses. University of Chicago Press; 1939.
2. Wandersman A, Nation M. Urban neighborhoods and mental health. Psychological contributions to understanding toxicity, resilience, and interventions. Am Psychol. 1998;53(6):647–56.
3. Evans GW, Wells NM, Moch A. Housing and mental health: a review of the evidence and a methodological and conceptual critique. J Soc Issues. 2003;59(3):475–500. https://doi.org/10.1111/1540-4560.00074.
4. Peen J, Schoevers RA, Beekman AT, Dekker J. The current status of urban-rural differences in psychiatric disorders. Acta Psychiatr Scand. 2010;121(2):84–93.
5. Miles R, Coutts C, Mohamadi A. Neighborhood urban form, social environment, and depression. J Urban Health. 2012;89(1):1–18. https://doi.org/10.1007/s11524-011-9621-2.
6. Gruebner O, Rapp MA, Adli M, Kluge U, Galea S, Heinz A. Cities and mental health. Dtsch Arztebl Int. 2017;114:121–7. https://doi.org/10.3238/arztebl.2017.0121.
7. Li J, Rose N. Urban social exclusion and mental health of China's rural-urban migrants – a review and call for research. Health Place. 2017;48:20–30. https://doi.org/10.1016/j.healthplace.2017.08.009.
8. Okkels N, Kristiansen CB, Munk-Jørgensen P, Sartorius N. Urban mental health. Curr Opin Psychiatry. 2018;31:258–64. https://doi.org/10.1097/YCO.0000000000000413.
9. Manning N. Sociology, biology and mechanisms in urban mental health. Soc Theory Health. 2018;17:1–22. https://doi.org/10.1057/s41285-018-00085-7.
10. Baumann PS, Söderström O, Abrahamyan Empson L, Söderström D, Codeluppi Z, Golay P, et al. Urban remediation: a new recovery-oriented strategy to manage urban stress after first-episode psychosis. Soc Psychiatry Psychiatr Epidemiol. 2019;55:273–83. https://doi.org/10.1007/s00127-019-01795-7.
11. Generaal E, Hoogendijk EO, Stam M, Henke CE, Rutters F, Oosterman M, et al. Neighbourhood characteristics, prevalence, and severity of depression: pooled analysis of eight Dutch cohort studies. Br J Psychiatry. 2019;2019:1–8. https://doi.org/10.1192/bjp.2019.100.
12. Lecic-Tosevski D. Is urban living good for mental health? Curr Opin Psychiatry. 2019;32(3):204–9. https://doi.org/10.1097/YCO.0000000000000489.
13. Ventriglio A, Torales J, Castaldelli-Maia JM, De Berardis D, Bhugra D. Urbanization and emerging mental health issues. CNS Spectr. 2020;2020:1–8. https://doi.org/10.1017/S1092852920001236.
14. D'Acci LS. Urbanicity mental costs valuation: a review and urban-societal planning consideration. Mind Soc. 2020;9:223–35. https://doi.org/10.1007/s11299-020-00235-3.
15. Mari J. Mental health in big cities. Editorial. Curr Opin Psychiatry. 2020;33(3):231–2. https://doi.org/10.1097/yco.0000000000000599.
16. Sampson L, Ettman CK, Galea S. Urbanization, urbanicity, and depression. Curr Opin Psychiatry. 2020;33(3):233–44. https://doi.org/10.1097/YCO.0000000000000588.
17. Litman TA. Urban sanity understanding urban mental health impacts and how to create saner. Happier Cities. 2021; https://vtpi.org/urban-sanity.pdf
18. Simmel J. The metropolis and mental life. Section 7 of the people, place, and space reader, 1903, p. 223–6.
19. Prindle RA. Health aspects of the urban environment. Public Health Rep. 1968;83(7):617–21. https://doi.org/10.2307/4593367.
20. Milgram S. The experience of living in cities. Science. 1970;167(3924):1461–8. https://doi.org/10.1126/science.167.3924.1461.
21. Proshansky HM. Urban stress. Experiments on noise and social stressors. David C. Glass and Jerome E. Singer. Academic Press, New York, 1972. xiv, 182 pp., illus. $8.75. Social Psychology. Science. 178(4067):1275A. https://doi.org/10.1126/science.178.4067.1275a.

22. Christmas JJ. Psychological stresses of urban living: new direction for mental health services in the inner city. J Natl Med Assoc. 1973;65(6):483.
23. Lazarus RS, Cohen JB. Environmental stress. Hum Behav Environ. 1977;1977:89–127. https://doi.org/10.1007/978-1-4684-0808-9_3.
24. Webb SD, Collette J. Rural-urban differences in the use of stress-alleviative drugs. Am J Sociol. 1977;83(3):700–7. https://doi.org/10.1086/226600.
25. Baum AS, Jerome EB, Carlene S. Stress and the environment. Soc Issues. 1981;37(1):4–35. https://doi.org/10.1111/j.1540-4560.1981.tb01056.x.
26. Cohen S, Evans GW, Stokols D, Krantz DS. Environmental stress and cognitive performance. In: Cohen S, Evans GW, Stokols D, Krantz DS, editors. Behaviour, health, and environmental stress. Springer: Berlin; 1986. p. 143–83.
27. Burton I. Factors in urban stress. J Sociol Soc Welf. 1990;17(1).
28. Lin N, Lai G. Urban stress in China. Soc Sci Med. 1995;41(8):1131–45. https://doi.org/10.1016/0277-9536(94)00426-t.
29. Haines MM, Stansfeld SA, Job RFS, Berglund B, Head J. Chronic aircraft noise exposure, stress responses, mental health and cognitive performance in school children. Psychol Med. 2001;31(2):265–77. https://doi.org/10.1017/S0033291701003282.
30. Jaffee KD, Liu GC, Canty-Mitchell J, Qi RA, Austin J, Swigonski N. Race, urban community stressors, and behavioral and emotional problems of children with special health care needs. Psychiatr Serv. 2005;56(1):63–9. https://doi.org/10.1176/appi.ps.56.1.63.
31. Miller KM, Phillips MH. Correlates of urban stress and mental health: the impact of social context on resilience. J Soc Distress Homeless. 2005;14(1–2):46–64. https://doi.org/10.1179/105307805807066301.
32. Suchday S, Kapur S, Ewart CK, Friedberg JP. Urban stress and health in developing countries: development and validation of a neighborhood stress index for India. Behav Med. 2006;32(3):77–86. https://doi.org/10.3200/bmed.32.3.77-86.
33. Quinn K, Kaufman JS, Siddiqi A, Yeatts KB. Stress and the city: housing stressors are associated with respiratory health among low socioeconomic status Chicago children. PLoS One. 2010;87(4):688–702. https://doi.org/10.1007/s11524-010-9465-1.
34. Adli M. Urban stress and mental health. Cities, health and well-being, Hong Kong; 2011.
35. Lederbogen F, Kirsch P, Haddad L, Streit F, Tost H, Schuch P, et al. City living and urban upbringing affect neural social stress processing in humans. Nature. 2011;474:498–501.
36. Seth P, Murray CC, Braxton ND, DiClemente RJ. The concrete jungle: city stress and substance abuse among young adult African American men. J Urban Health. 2012;90(2):307–13. https://doi.org/10.1007/s11524-012-9716-4.
37. Rishi P, Khuntia G. Urban environmental stress and behavioral adaptation in Bhopal City of India. Urban Stud Res. 2012;2012:1–9. https://doi.org/10.1155/2012/635061.
38. Lederbogen F, Haddad L, Meyer-Lindenberg A. Urban social stress – risk factor for mental disorders. The case of schizophrenia. Environ Pollut. 2013;183:2–6. https://doi.org/10.1016/j.envpol.2013.05.046.
39. Steinheuser V, Ackermann K, Pia A, Lars S. Stress and the city. Psychosom Med. 2014;76(9):678–85. https://doi.org/10.1097/PSY.0000000000000113.
40. Knöll M, Neuheuser K, Vogt J, Rudolph-Cleff A. Einflussfaktoren der gebauten Umwelt auf wahrgenommene Aufenthaltsqualität bei der Nutzung städtischer Räume. Umweltpsychologie. 2014;18:84–102. https://www.researchgate.net/publication/270759025
41. Freeman D, Emsley R, Dunn G, Fowler D, Bebbington P, Kuipers E, et al. The stress of the street for patients with persecutory delusions: a test of the symptomatic and psychological effects of going outside into a busy urban area. Schizophr Bull. 2015;41(4):971–9. https://doi.org/10.1093/schbul/sbu173.
42. Willie TC, Powell A, Kershaw T. Stress in the city: influence of urban social stress and violence on pregnancy and postpartum quality of life among adolescent and young mothers. J Urban Health. 2016;93(1):19–35. https://doi.org/10.1007/s11524-015-0021-x.

43. Adli M, Berger M, Brakemeier E-L, Engel L, Fingerhut J, Hehl R, et al. Neurourbanistik – ein methodischer Schulterschluss zwischen Stadtplanung und Neurowissenschaften. Die Psychiatrie. 2016;13:70–8.
44. Knöll M, Neuheuser K, Cleff T, Rudolph-Cleff A. A tool to predict perceived urban stress in open public spaces. Environ Plan B Urban Anal City Sci. 2017;45:797–813. https://doi.org/10.1177/0265813516686971.
45. Mubi Brighenti A, Pavoni A. City of unpleasant feelings. Stress, comfort and animosity in urban life. Soc Cult Geogr. 2017;20:1–20. https://doi.org/10.1080/14649365.2017.1355065.
46. Söderström O, Söderström D, Codeluppi Z, Abrahamyan Empson L, Conus P. Emplacing recovery: how persons diagnosed with psychosis handle stress in cities. Psychosis. 2017;9:322–9. https://doi.org/10.1080/17522439.2017.1344296.
47. Elsamahy EM, Abd El-Fattah R. Designing non-stressed psychological public spaces. BAU J Health Well-Being. 2018;2018:121–32.
48. Mukherjee A, Agrawal M. The influence of urban stress factors on responses of ground cover vegetation. Environ Sci Pollut Res. 2018;25:36194–206. https://doi.org/10.1007/s11356-018-3437-5.
49. Li J, Liu Z. Housing stress and mental health of migrant populations in urban China. Cities. 2018;81:172–9. https://doi.org/10.1016/j.cities.2018.04.006.
50. Chrisinger BW, King AC. Stress experiences in neighborhood and social environments (SENSE): a pilot study to integrate the quantified self with citizen science to improve the built environment and health. Int J Health Geogr. 2018;17(1):17. https://doi.org/10.1186/s12942-018-0140-1.
51. Fett AJ, Lemmers-Jansen ILJ, Krabbendam L. Psychosis and urbanicity. Curr Opin Psychiatry. 2019;32(3):232–41. https://doi.org/10.1097/yco.0000000000000486.
52. Kyriakou K, Resch B. Spatial analysis of moments of stress derived from wearable sensor data. Adv Cartogr GIScience Int Cartogr Assoc. 2019;2:9. https://doi.org/10.5194/ica-adv-2-9-2019.
53. Meloni A, Fornara F, Carrus G. Predicting pro-environmental behaviors in the urban context: the direct or moderated effect of urban stress, city identity, and worldviews. Cities. 2019;88:83–90. https://doi.org/10.1016/j.cities.2019.01.001.
54. Werner C, Resch B, Loidl M. Evaluating urban bicycle infrastructures through intersubjectivity of stress sensations derived from physiological measurements. ISPRS Int J Geo Inf. 2019;8(6):265. https://doi.org/10.3390/ijgi8060265.
55. Birenboim A, Dijst M, Scheepers FE, Poelman MP, Helbich M. Wearables and location tracking technologies for mental-state sensing in outdoor environments. Prof Geogr. 2019;71:449–61. https://doi.org/10.1080/00330124.2018.1547978.
56. Pykett J, Osborne T, Resch B. From urban stress to neurourbanism: how should we research city well-being? Ann Am Assoc Geogr. 2020;2020:1–16. https://doi.org/10.1080/24694452.2020.1736982.
57. Pykett J, Chrisinger B, Kyriakou K, Osborne T, Resch B, Stathi A, et al. Developing a Citizen Social Science approach to understand urban stress and promote wellbeing in urban communities. Palgrave Commun. 2020;6:85. https://doi.org/10.1057/s41599-020-0460-1.
58. Adli M, Schondorf J. Macht uns die Stadt krank. Wirkung von Stadtstress auf Emotionen, Verhalten und psychische Gesundheit; Does the city make us ill? The effect of urban stress on emotions, behavior, and mental health. Bundesgesundheitsbl. 2020;63:979–86. https://doi.org/10.1007/s00103-020-03185-w.
59. Vargas T, Conley RE, Mittal VA. Chronic stress, structural exposures and neurobiological mechanisms: a stimulation, discrepancy and deprivation model of psychosis. In: Clow A, Smyth N, editors. International review of neurobiology; 2020. p. 41–69. https://doi.org/10.1016/bs.irn.2019.11.004.
60. Shannon MM, Clougherty JE, McCarthy C, Elovitz MA, Nguemeni Tiako MJ, Melly SJ, et al. Neighborhood violent crime and perceived stress in pregnancy. Int J Environ Res Public Health. 2020;17(15):5585. https://doi.org/10.3390/ijerph17155585.

61. Hernandez DC, Daundasekara SS, Zvolensky MJ, Reitzel LR, Maria DS, Alexander AC, et al. Urban stress indirectly influences psychological symptoms through its association with distress tolerance and perceived social support among adults experiencing homelessness. Int J Environ Res Public Health. 2020;17(15):5301. https://doi.org/10.3390/ijerph17155301.
62. Evans BE, Huizink AC, Greaves-Lord K, Tulen JHM, Roelofs K, van der Ende J, Santana GL. Urbanicity, biological stress system functioning and mental health in adolescents. PLoS One. 2020;15(3):e0228659. https://doi.org/10.1371/journal.pone.0228659.
63. Dykas MJ, Goplen J, Ewart CK, Gump BB. Early adolescents' risk taking propensity, urban stress, and affiliation with risky peers. J Early Adolesc. 2021;41(5):683–99. https://doi.org/10.1177/0272431620939192.
64. Buttazzoni A, Doherty S, Minaker L. How do urban environments affect young people's mental health? A novel conceptual framework to bridge public health, planning, and neurourbanism. Public Health Rep. 2021;137:48–61. https://doi.org/10.1177/0033354920982088.
65. Knox City Council. Knox mental health action plan 2021–2025. 2021. https://www.knox.vic.gov.au.
66. Ararat City Council. Ararat City municipal public health and wellbeing plan 2013–2017. 2013. https://www. Ararat.vic.gov.au.
67. Moreland City Council. Moreland municipal public health and wellbeing plan 2017–2021. 2017. https://www.moreland.vic.gov.au.
68. Casey City Council. Municipal public health and wellbeing plan 2017–2021. 2017. https://www.casey.vic.gov.au.
69. Northern Grampians City Council. Northern Grampians municipal public health and wellbeing plan 2017–2021. 2017. https://nla.gov.au.
70. Victoria State Government. Victorian public health and wellbeing plan (2011–2015). 2011. https://www2.health.vic.gov.au.
71. Victoria State Government. Victorian public health and wellbeing plan (2015–2019). 2015. https://www2.health.vic.gov.au.
72. Victoria State Government. Victorian public health and wellbeing plan (2019–2023). 2019. https://www2.health.vic.gov.au.

Chapter 7
Presenting the Theoretical Framework of Stress Relief Urban Planning

Abstract This chapter describes the concept of stress relief urban planning first. Then, according to the identified stressful factors, indicators have been identified, and relationships between them are defined using content analysis. Finally, the theoretical framework and conceptual model of this planning are presented.

After introducing the general indicators of stress-relief urban planning, due to the very low frequencies of some indicators and the difficulty of drawing a conceptual model due to the great number of indicators, the interrelationships between the indicators were examined using the Maxqda software and analyzing the content of relevant research, and it was tried to identify the most important indicators considering their interrelationships and frequencies.

How the dimensions of stress-relief urban planning interact with each other is very important. For this purpose, after examining the relationships between the effective indicators in this section using the (Maxqda) software, the relationships between the dimensions abovementioned were examined.

In this chapter, after identifying the relationship between urban mental health and urban stress, the general research indicators are presented in the form of the theoretical framework and the relationships between them are shown. Moreover, according to the relationships presented in the previous sections and the most important and influential general research indicators, the research conceptual model is presented. According to this figure, urban mental health and urban stress mutually influence each other (directly and indirectly). The indicators extracted from theoretical foundations are classified into two groups.

Keywords Urban stress · Neurourbanism · Stress-relief urban planning

S. Jalilisadrabad et al., *Stress Relief Urban Planning*,
https://doi.org/10.1007/978-981-99-4202-2_7

7.1 Introduction

This chapter describes the concept of stress relief urban planning first. Then, according to the identified stressful factors, indicators have been identified, and relationships between them are defined using content analysis. Finally, the theoretical framework and conceptual model of this planning are presented.

7.2 Neurourbanism

Epidemiological research has highlighted the prevalence of mental diseases and stress among urbanites, as mentioned in the previous chapters [1]. The study of the connection between the human brain, urban density, urban landscapes, and architectural forms has been categorised into the fields of neuroarchitecture, neurourbanism, and psychophysiological research due to the significance of this subject in cities [2]. A mental health strategy for cities called neurourbanism places a strong emphasis on the idea of prevention. It is a strategy that links urban planning and public mental health to improve urban environments [3].

The series of international and interdisciplinary urban brain workshops hosted in London since 2013 was one of the most basic measures and effective approaches to urban mental health, one of the results of which is a call for experimental studies in the field of Neuropolis. After holding these workshops, the city was examined as a psychological phenomenon in addition to a geographical, spatial, political, commercial, and economic reality [4]. Then, in 2019, the interdisciplinary forum for neurourbanistics led by the medical department of Berlin University and consisting of neuroscientists, psychiatrists, psychologists, architects, urban planners, sociologists, geographers, and philosophers published the "Charta of Neurourbanism" which summarizes research priorities and initial recommendations for action for psychologically healthier cities [5]. This charter paves the way towards psychoanalysis and modern imagination of the dynamic relationships of the urban environment [6] and provides a valuable insight into the complex interaction between the city and the human psyche. However, some recommendations of this charter such as density and aesthetics, are very ambiguous [7].

To respond to the goals of neuro urbanism, it is necessary to identify the research challenges of this field [8]. Table 7.1 introduces these challenges.

Table 7.1 Introducing the research challenges of neuro urbanism [8]

Research challenges of neuro urbanism	The first issue: the interaction between humans and the urban environment
	1. Exploring the influence of the built environment on psychological well-being (the influence of the characteristics of the built environment on psychological well-being). 2. Investigating the impact of designing social settings on psychological well-being (the impact of urban living space on the mental health of city residents, including the impact of urban and neighborhood planning on the mental health of individuals and communities, social support structures, social integration, subjective experience of security within urban). 3. Investigating the interaction between urban living space, social behavior, and self-efficacy experience (urban planning affects the processes of participation, acquisition, and fragmentation of urban population through density, compaction, spatial separation (public, private, semi-public), spatial granularity, and permeability).
	The second issue: characteristics of stress in the county
	1. Exploring urban stressors and their facilitators. 2. Identifying the population influenced by "urban stress" (immigrants, the elderly, the youth, children, women, etc.).
	The third issue: socialization, prevention, and treatment
	1. Investigating the influence of architecture and urban planning on the social and emotional maturation processes of children and adolescents (15 years old). 2. Developing the concepts of prevention and treatment for "urban diseases". 3. Designing action plans to promote mental health in cities and municipalities.

7.3 Stress-Relief Urban Planning (Neuro-Urban Planning)

In order to address the impact of urban living on mental health, neuro-urban planning focuses on identifying high-risk populations (such as migrants) and defining urban stressors. Therefore, it is important to accurately identify urban stressors and those variables that turn urban stress into chronic stress in order to apply neuro-urban design. The name "neuro-urbanism" has been proposed to describe this interdisciplinary approach, which must integrate architecture, urban planning, neurology, and medicine. Creating surroundings that boost urban residents' resilience and mental health is the aim of neuro-urban planning. This planning doesn't aim to remove people from urban environments or to condemn the city. Because cities offer more advantages to their residents than their disadvantages. Also, there are more opportunities for social participation, education, well-being, and personal development in the city than in its suburbs. Rather, it aims to develop urban planning including a neuro-urbanist perspective and seeking to reduce urban stressors [8]. Neuro-urbanism, as a novel approach, can help to respond appropriately and effectively to the challenges of mental health in an urban world [8]. The charta of neuro urbanism proposes solutions in nine areas to promote mental health and reduce urban stress, as shown in Table 7.2:

Table 7.2 Introducing the solutions presented by the "Charta of Neurourbanism" [5, 8]

Aspect	Description
Density	Density is one of the advantages of urban life. However, it can lead to urban stress. Social density is positive when a person does not feel unable and has control over his surroundings. High density and low environmental mastery increase the probability of experiencing chronic stress.
Interpersonal relationships	Social loneliness and social isolation are among the main causes of urban stress, and the city should strengthen the motivation to establish social interactions among its residents. Urban planning prerequisites for this include sidewalks, parks, open spaces, etc., and vulnerable populations such as immigrants, the elderly, the sick, the poor, etc. should be given special consideration.
Encountering the public	The design of public space provides a framework for urbanites to meet each other. These interactions form social support structures.
Diversity	Urban diversity is an important prerequisite for socialization and mental health processes since it helps to acquire social skills. It plays a role in the development of social diversity and the implementation of an open city.
Aesthetics	The aesthetic aspects of a city affect our emotions, and this perception depends on four factors: sufficient complexity of the landscape, a high degree of coherence, easy comprehension, and a certain degree of mystery that arouses curiosity and the need for exploration.
Avoiding segregation	Urban neighborhoods should include different social milieus living together side by side and characterized by their neighborhoods. Identification with one's neighborhood is a community-building factor that promotes the social cohesion and sense of belonging of old and new residents. Also, Changes in the cityscape must not lead to the expulsion of the "traditional".
Mobility	Active mobility in the city promotes meaningful social connections in the city and enhances a person's feeling of control over the environment. The longer and more complicated daily routes, and the more monofunctional the destinations, the more stressful a person experiences.
Facilitating participation	Good urban governance encourages political, administrative, economic, and cultural participation and empowers them, and as a result, increases their self-efficacy and the experience of environmental mastery.
Culture	Cultural institutions and cultural sites are urban meeting places. They promote a sense of belonging and reduce social isolation.

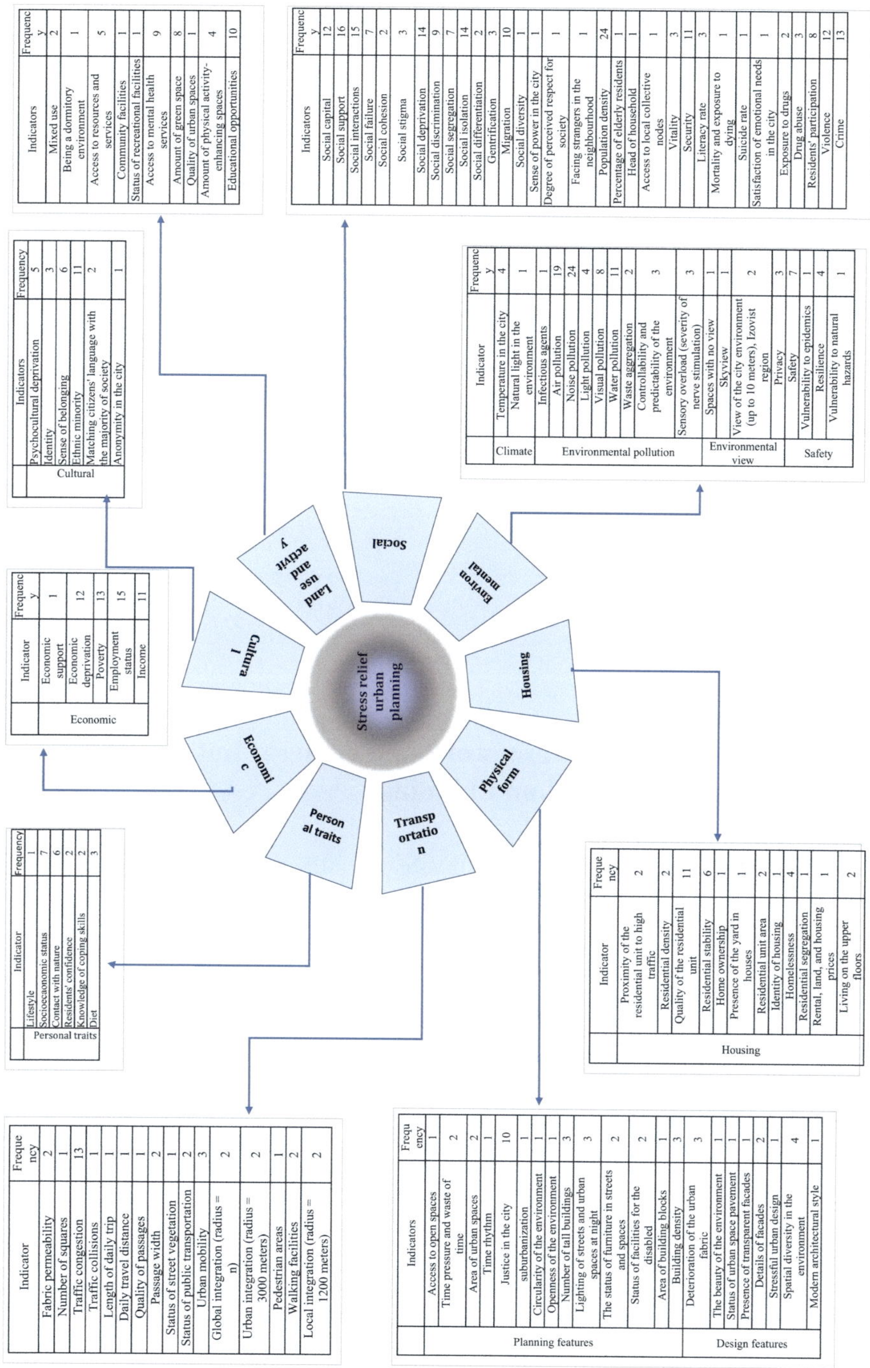

Fig. 7.1 The theoretical framework of stress-relief urban planning

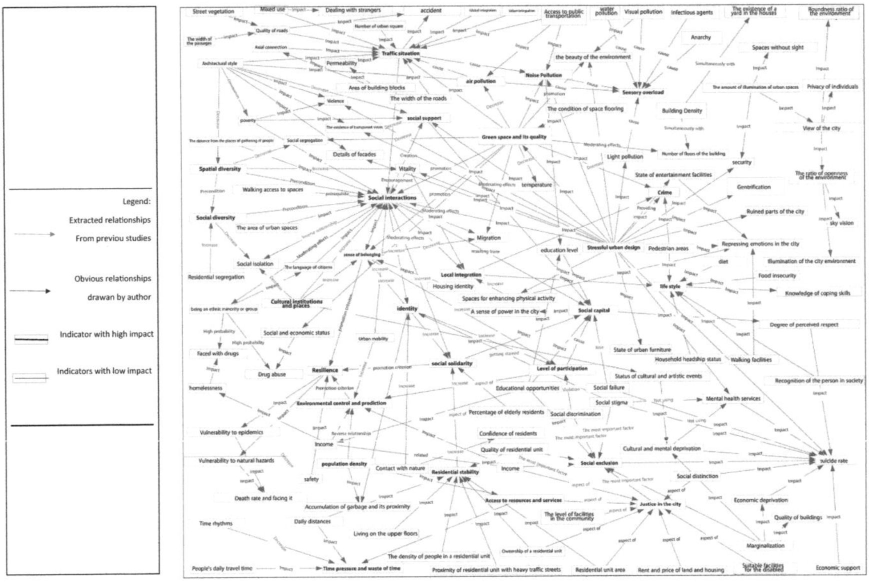

Fig. 7.2 The relationships between stress-relief urban planning indicators

7.4 The Theoretical Framework and General Indicators of Stress-Relief Urban Planning

In this section, considering the urban stressors identified in Table 3.2 and the summary of successful global experiences in Table 6.3, it was attempted to develop general indicators affecting stress-relief urban planning, as listed in Fig. 7.1. Also, the frequencies of these indicators are presented according to the summary of these tables.

7.5 Examining the Relationships Between Stress-Relief Urban Planning Indicators

After introducing the general indicators of stress-relief urban planning in Fig. 7.1, due to the very low frequencies of some indicators and the difficulty of drawing a conceptual model due to the great number of indicators, the interrelationships between the indicators were examined using the Maxqda software and analyzing the content of relevant research, and it was tried to identify the most important indicators considering their interrelationships and frequencies. For this purpose, Fig. 7.2 shows the interrelationships between the indicators. According to this figure, the indicators of stressful urban design, modern architectural style, green spaces, and the accessibility and quality of green spaces were identified as the most effective indicators. Also, indicators of social interactions, social capital, crime, noise pollution, sensory overload, justice in the city, social exclusion, suicide rate, environmental control and prediction, lifestyle, residential stability, level of participation, and traffic density were identified as the most influenced stress-relief urban planning indicators.

It should be noted that in the figure, the relationships shown in blue were extracted from previous studies, while those in red are obvious relationships drawn by the authors. All these relationships are direct and it was not possible to show indirect relationships in the figure. However, it is possible to discover indirect relationships from direct ones in the figure. For example:

- Spatial diversity in the environment affects local integration through vitality.
- Contact with nature strengthens the sense of belonging through the promotion of identity.
- The rent and prices of land and housing, as aspects of urban justice, affect social deprivation.
- Being an ethnic minority influences the citizens' social interactions by influencing their language.

Table 7.3 The content of relationships between indicators

Item	Content of relationships between indicators	Reference
Urbanites face the stress induced by time pressure and waste of more time, which can be reduced by urban planning and social and economic daily lifestyles, such as telecommuting plus flexible working hours, nationally reducing weekly working hours, waiting times at stations and public transportation, the distance between work and living environment and services, etc.	Time rhythms affect time pressure and waste of time	[9]
	Length of daily travel affects time pressure and waste of time	
	Greater distances affect time pressure and waste time	
	Access to resources and services affects time pressure and waste time	
The plan focused on the gardening of flowers and edible vegetables, resulting in promoted self-confidence, revitalized neighborhood, increased sociability, reduced sabotage, improved abandoned land, revitalized public buildings, reduced urban stress, and improved sense of belonging and identity among lower-class citizens.	Contact with nature promotes residents' confidence	[10]
	Green space and access to it reduce crime	
	Green space and access to it promote a sense of belonging	
	Green space and access to it promote identity	
	Green space and access to it moderates the effects of lower social and economic status	
	Green space and access to it enhance social interactions	

(continued)

Table 7.3 (continued)

Item	Content of relationships between indicators	Reference
Urban congestion (as opposed to sprawl) has been associated with better mental health as it provides better access to resources, such as parks, playgrounds, health, and social care.	Urban congestion can enhance access to resources and services	[11]
High building density is also one of the important causes of urban stress due to the lack of space, the mass of the building, and the very great number of floors.	High building density is in line with the number of floors	[12]
	The high density of the building is in line with the presence of the yard in houses	
The resilience promotion strategies can minimize exposure to social stress, promote social cohesion and a sense of belonging, enable allocation processes, and enhance the experience of dominance over the environment.	Social cohesion promotes resilience	[5]
	A sense of belonging promotes resilience	
	Dominance over the environment promotes resilience	
Instead of staying in the environment and trying to improve it, most people look for ways to physically escape from it, and the best solution to it is to promote a sense of belonging against this physical escape.	A sense of belonging reduces migration	[13]
When communities have positive social interactions, neighborhood pride, interest, and cohesion are improved and the potential for coping with the cumulative elimination factors associated with living in urban neighborhoods is reduced.	Social interactions promote social cohesion	[13]
The promotion of social support networks, such as peer support, civic engagement in local institutions as volunteers, efforts to improve the quality of education and literacy, social cohesion, and social control are the most important strategies to promote social capital in the neighborhood.	Social support is the most important solution to promote social capital	[14]
	Social interactions are the most important solution to promoting social capital	
	Quality of education is the most important way to promote social capital	
	Improving the level of literacy is the most important way to promote social capital	
	Social cohesion is the most important way to promote social capital	

Table 7.3 (continued)

Item	Content of relationships between indicators	Reference
People living in pro-community and pedestrian areas have reported lower levels of mental distress, lower crime rates, lower obesity rates, and lower rates of chronic illness. Providing vibrant and sociable environments that are clean and pleasant; promoting walking and social interaction between people; providing sustainable public transportation, sports-encouraging environments, access to drinking fountains, and sitting places; and extensively connecting local streets are effective solutions to promote local integration.	Pedestrian areas reduce crime	[15]
	Walking facilities reduce crime	
	Local integration reduces crime	
	Vitality encourages social interactions	
	Vitality promotes local integration	
	Physical activity-enhancing spaces are an effective way to promote local integration	
Social interactions among the residents of the neighborhood when walking, the existence of parks and green spaces, and the physical activity resulting from walking improve citizens' mental health.	Local integration promotes social interactions	[16]
	The presence of physical activity-enhancing spaces promotes local integration	
The nature of modern urbanization may have knock-on consequences for mental health by influencing stressors and adverse life events, such as crowded and polluted environments, poverty and dependence on the cash economy, high levels of violence declined social support and the creation of lifeless environments. Therefore, in planning for a city, it is required to consider a sufficient number of natural settings such as pollution buffers (noise, dust, etc.) and provide a beautiful space to improve the quality of the surrounding environment.	Modern architectural style influences air pollution	[17]
	Modern architectural style influences poverty	
	Modern architectural style influences violence	
	Modern architectural style influences social support	
	Modern architectural style influences the details of the facades	
	Green spaces are effective in promoting the beauty of the environment	
	Green space affects noise	
Repetitive patterns in modern architecture may hurt, and harm mental health by affecting the sense of sight and neural processing.	Modern architecture affects repetitive patterns	[18]
Promoting justice in the urban environment in various aspects, such as the distribution of resources and services may further promote mental health in urban areas.	Proper distribution of services is an aspect of justice in the city	[11]

(continued)

Table 7.3 (continued)

Item	Content of relationships between indicators	Reference
A diverse urban space is an important prerequisite for the processes of socialization and mental health since it helps to acquire social skills. It contributes to the development of social diversity and the creation of an open city. While the diversity of urban space is an important factor playing a role in its vitality, current developments have a strong tendency to homogenize neighborhoods. Fragmenting the city into homogeneous neighborhoods disrupts the dynamics of the city as an open system. Also, a lack of sociocultural diversity, in turn, can lead to the reduction of social skills and the promotion of social isolation and conflict in the city.	Spatial diversity is a prerequisite for social diversity	[8]
	Spatial diversity is a prerequisite for social interactions	
	Spatial diversity brings vitality to the urban environment	
	Social diversity reduces social isolation	
Housing planning for low-income groups is a new approach to ending the chronic homelessness of low-income people who are more likely to be prone to mental illness and drug abuse.	Socioeconomic status affects drug abuse	[19]
	Income influences homelessness	
	Homelessness influences drug abuse	
The strategy of mixedly leasing out housing to rich and deprived residents or constructing apartments containing both private and rental units can be effective in promoting mental health by creating social diversity.	The lack of residential segregation promotes social diversity	[20]
Residential stability in the neighborhood and the concentration of the elderly, regardless of economic deprivation indicators, is an aspect of social cohesion associated with depression and stress.	Residential stability is an aspect of social cohesion	[16]
	The high percentage of the elderly is an aspect of social cohesion	
The urban design may promote mental health through these places within the framework of the GAPS (GAPS: Green places, Active places, Prosocial places, and Safe places) strategy.	Urban design affects green spaces	[21]
	Urban design affects physical activity-enhancing places	
	Urban design affects security	
	Urban design affects social interactions	
Urban green areas improve air quality, reduce noise pollution, improve traffic, increase social interaction, and reduce stress.	Green spaces improve air quality	[19]
	Green spaces reduce noise pollution	
	Green spaces improve traffic	
	Green spaces enhance social interactions	
The availability of cycling paths and public transportation, including the metro, can reduce car use, which is associated with more traffic, noise, and air pollution, thereby reducing stress.	Proper access to public transport reduces traffic	[21]
	Proper access to public transport reduces noise pollution	
	Proper access to public transport reduces air pollution	

Table 7.3 (continued)

Item	Content of relationships between indicators	Reference
Active mobility in the city promotes significant social communication in the city and enhances a sense of personal control over the environment.	Urban mobility promotes social interactions	[8]
	Urban mobility enhances one's control over the environment	
Stress management techniques (e.g., relaxation, meditation, sports activities), trauma therapy, promoting urban group walking, use of new technologies (e.g., instantaneous ecological interventions, virtual reality, mobile applications) can be helpful in this area.	Social interactions enhance the impact of local integration	[22]
Living in neighborhoods with a higher density of private cars was associated with more stress symptoms due to chronic noise.	Traffic congestion causes noise pollution	[16]
Social deprivation reduces the mental health of immigrants, and the most important factors causing it is limited access to full employment rights, the experience of social stigma, discrimination, and injustice.	Employment is one of the most important factors of social deprivation	[18]
	Social stigma is one of the most important factors in social deprivation	
	Social discrimination is one of the most important factors of social deprivation	
	Injustice is one of the most important factors of social deprivation	
Chronic exposure to aircraft noise is associated with impaired reading comprehension and high levels of noise, but not mental health problems in children, and factors, such as social class and deprivation play a mediating role here.	Noise pollution disrupts education	[23]
African American men living in a stressful urban environment are at increased risk of being exposed to and using drugs. Culturally competent public health interventions to control drug use should address psychological factors, such as stress and neighborhood violence.	Being of an ethnic or group minority leads to greater exposure to drug abuse	[24]
	Being an ethnic or group minority increases the likelihood of drug abuse	
	Violence needs to be investigated to address drug abuse	
The results show that both urban stress and the affirmation of sustainable worldviews are significant positive predictors of eco-friendly behavior. City identity moderates the relationship between urban stress and the willingness to pay for green energy and generate no waste, respectively.	Identity moderates excessive waste accumulation	[25]

(continued)

Table 7.3 (continued)

Item	Content of relationships between indicators	Reference
Changing residential use to commercial and office uses would increase encounters with strangers in the neighborhood.	Land use is effective in encountering strangers	[26]
One of the most tangible consequences of land use change is traffic problems.	Land-use influences traffic congestion	[26]
The number of people and how they live affects environmental conditions through the use of natural resources and waste generation.	Population density can affect mental health through waste generation	[27]
Environmental stressors in cities, such as traffic, can cause stress, which often appears in the form of physical disturbance, mental illness, and reduced social interaction.	Traffic congestion reduces social interactions	[17]
Circularity is obtained by dividing the isovist area by the perimeter squared.	The adequate relative view influences circularity	[28]
The ratio of openness refers to the balance between the closed and open edges of an isovist and is related to its interestingness and complexity.	The adequate relative view influences the openness of space	[12]
When secondary stimuli, such as sound, light, etc. cannot be cut off and cause distraction, irritation, and confusion, the person is subjected to sensory overload.	Pollutions cause sensory overload if left uncontrolled	[29]
Social capital refers to the collective capabilities resulting from social networks.	Social interactions result from social capital	[30]
Social capital refers to the commitments, interactions, participation, relationships, and interests that unite people in a community.	Social participation creates social capital	[31]
Social support is supportive interactions among people against the health consequences and stressors of life.	Social interactions create social support	[32]
Social failure is the feeling of failure in struggle and loss of social status or failure in access to social resources.	Social failure causes a loss of social capital	[33]
Social cohesion is a sense of connection, desire, and tendency between individuals and refers to a sense of mutual responsibility between one or more individuals or groups.	Social cohesion triggers social interactions	[34]
Social stigma is the tarnishing of a person's social identity, which discredits and demeans him.	Social stigma diminishes identity	[35]
Social deprivation includes different levels and aspects, such as access to employment, education, housing, skills, and private and public spaces. People who do not have these cases and do not have proper citizenship rights are called socially deprived.	Lack of access to employment leads to social deprivation	[36]
	Lack of access to education leads to social deprivation	
	Lack of access to quality housing leads to social deprivation	
Social discrimination is an act that intentionally violates social participation or human rights for a group of people.	Social discrimination violates social participation	[37]

Table 7.3 (continued)

Item	Content of relationships between indicators	Reference
Social isolation refers to the lack or weakness of a person's relationships with other individuals and groups in society so that the person feels not belong to society.	Social relationships affect social isolation	[38]
	Social relationships affect the sense of belonging	
Social density is positive when a person does not feel helpless and has control over their environment, but at high density and low environmental dominance, the likelihood of experiencing chronic stress increases. Social loneliness and isolation are the main causes of urban stress and the city should strengthen the motivation for social interactions among its residents. Prerequisites for urban planning for this are sidewalks, parks, and open spaces and at-risk populations, such as immigrants, the elderly, the sick, and the poor should be given priority. By designing and proposing public space, a framework can be provided for urbanites to meet with each other. It is such interactions that create the structure of social support. A diverse urban space, in terms of helping to acquire social skills, is an important prerequisite for the processes of socialization and mental health, contributing to the development of social diversity and the creation of an open city. The aesthetic aspects of a city affect our emotions, and this perception depends on four factors: sufficient complexity of the landscape, high coherence, easy readability, and a certain degree of mystery that arouses curiosity and the need to explore. Urban neighborhoods should include different social environments that live together and are known for their neighborhoods. Identifying with your neighborhood is a community-building factor that enhances social cohesion and a sense of belonging among new and old residents. Also, changes in the urban landscape should not lead to the dismissal of veterans. Active mobility in the city promotes meaningful social communication in the city and promotes a sense of personal control over the environment. The later the daily distances end, the more complex and the more functional the single-purpose goals, and the more stress the person experiences. Good urban governance encourages political, administrative, economic, cultural, and empowerment participation of citizens, thereby increasing their self-efficacy and environmental experience. Cultural institutions and places are the meeting place of the city, which promote a sense of belonging and reduce social isolation.	Population density reduces the controllability and predictability of the environment	[8]
	Access to open spaces is a prerequisite for social interaction	
	Social interactions create the structure of social support	
	Social diversity is a precondition for social interactions	
	Spatial diversity leads to social diversity	
	Identity strengthens social cohesion	
	Identity strengthens the sense of belonging	
	Urban mobility promotes social interactions	
	Urban mobility promotes the controllability and predictability of the environment.	
	Social participation enhances the controllability and predictability of the environment.	
	Income influences the controllability and predictability of the environment.	
	Employment influences the controllability and predictability of the environment.	
	Cultural institutions and places enhance social interactions.	
	Cultural institutions and places reduce social isolation	
	Cultural institutions and places increase the sense of belonging	

(continued)

Table 7.3 (continued)

Item	Content of relationships between indicators	Reference
Workshops also promote the identity and sense of belonging to the city by fostering dialogue and expanding the social relations of individuals, especially immigrants and ethnic minorities, and ultimately promote citizen participation.	Social relationships promote identity	[39]
	Social relationships promote a sense of belonging	
	Identity promotes social participation	
	A sense of belonging promotes social participation	
	Social relations moderate the effects of migration	
	Social relations moderate the effects of being an ethnic or group minority	
Governmental and non-governmental organizations can play an important role in creating services and fostering a culture of optimal use through political, religious, and academic institutions.	Psychocultural deprivation prevents the use of psychological services	[40]
Research has shown that mental health services are available or inadequate in many urban environments, or are used because healthcare providers do not understand cultural differences. Citizens are also afraid of the stigma associated with mental illness, and insufficient insurance coverage is used, which is not placed optimally.	Social stigma can lead to the non-use of psychological services	[40]
Research has shown that mental health services are available or inadequate in many urban environments, or are used because healthcare providers do not understand cultural differences. Citizens are also afraid of the stigma associated with mental illness, and insufficient insurance coverage is used, which is not placed optimally.	Traffic congestion is caused by air pollution	[21]
	Green space and access to it reduce air pollution	
Green spaces reduce the effects of islands of urban heat and heat stress and can mitigate the stressful effects of tall buildings.	Green space and access to it moderate the effects of tall buildings	[11]
	Green space and access to it reduce the temperature of the city (e.g., effects of heat islands)	
Access to green space also moderates the negative and stressful aspects of migration, and migration to greener urban areas has been associated with sustained mental health improvements. Other benefits of green space include encouraging physical activity and promoting social relationships.	Green space and access to it moderate the effects of migration	[41]
	Green space and access to it promote social interactions	

Table 7.3 (continued)

Item	Content of relationships between indicators	Reference
Encouraging environmental diversity (e.g., a natural environment consisting of trees, plants, grasses, and species richness), especially in cities facing land and resource scarcity will reduce the gap between areas with high and low economic and social status.	Green space reduces the social segregation caused by the economic inequality	[20]
	Spatial diversity reduces the social segregation caused by the economic inequality	
The design of the built environment through physical stimuli (e.g., form, color, texture, sound, and light) has a significant effect on emotions, cognition, behavior, and ultimately psychological well-being.	Urban design affects noise pollution	[8]
	Urban design affects light pollution	
Urban design affects our perception by influencing the aesthetic aspects of a city, and this perception depends on four factors sufficient landscape complexity, high coherence, easy readability, and a certain degree of mystery that arouses curiosity and the need to explore.	Urban design affects the beauty of the environment	[8]
	Visual pollution affects the aesthetic aspects	
Urban design is a factor promoting mental health and urban stress because it may provide some places for recreational activities and relaxation; promote social support and security; and facilitate access to health care.	The urban design can provide leisure facilities	[21]
	Urban design promotes social support	
	The urban design promotes security	
	The urban design can facilitate access to mental health services	
The urban design may also affect crime and violence rates.	The urban design influences crime	[42]
	The urban design influences violence	
Urban furniture also has a great impact on mental health, so its proper design and location are very important.	Urban design affects the condition of urban furniture	[43]
Other factors affecting mental health in urban design are unsightly and heterogeneous views, and beauty, attractiveness, purity, and compatibility of views with local and cultural factors can be effective steps in promoting mental health.	Urban design influences landscapes	[44]
The use of warm colors in the urban environment induces a sense of joy, vibrancy, and movement, while the use of cold colors causes passivity, stillness, inactivity, and sadness.	Urban design affects vitality	[45]
Urban design can control suicide, which is one of the consequences of mental illness, by using strategies such as the use of physical barriers in buildings, stairs, railways, and subways.	The urban design affects the suicide rate	[21]

(continued)

- Suburbanization affects the suicide rate through the creation of economic deprivation.
- Homeownership influences social cohesion by affecting residential stability.
- The extent of population density affects resilience through its influence on the control and prediction of the environment.
- Residential segregation affects social interactions by reducing social diversity.
- The proximity of the residential unit to the high-traffic streets influences social cohesion through its impact on residential stability.

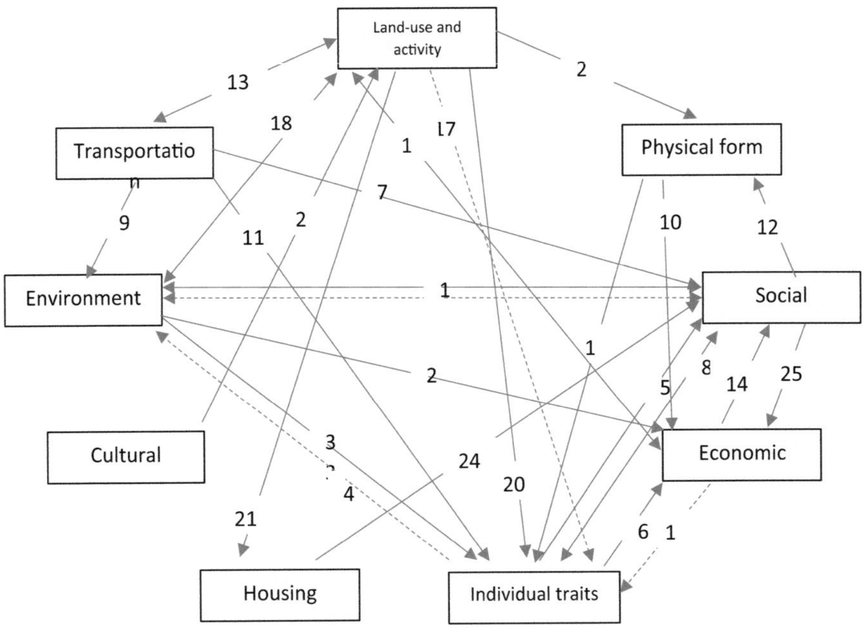

Fig. 7.3 The relationships between stress-relief urban planning dimensions

Table 7.4 The references from which the relationships shown in Fig. 7.3 were extracted

Relationship	Item	Direction of relationship	How the relationship is?	Reference
1	The relationship between environmental and social dimensions is shown in the figure.	Direct and indirect	Mutual effect	[46]
	Some experts have related environmental stressors to social factors.	Direct	Being related	[25]
	The increase in urban population density leads to the deterioration of the quality of the urban environment.	Direct	Effective	[47]
	The number of people and their lifestyles affect the environment through the use of natural resources and waste production.	Indirect	Effective	[27]
2	The relationship between environmental and economic dimensions is shown in the figure.	Direct and indirect	Effective	[46]
3	The relationship between the environmental dimension and individual traits is shown in the figure.	Direct and indirect	Effective	[46]
	Emotional understanding and evaluation of the environment affect the person's daily behavior and decisions in the space.	Direct	Effective	[48]
	The environment influences people's behavior, mood, cognitive performance, physical health, and psychological well-being.	Direct	Effective	[17]
4	People's lifestyles affect the environment through the use of natural resources and waste production.	Indirect	Effective	[27]
5	People's mental health has profound effects on individuals, communities, and economies.	Direct	Effective	[49]
6	People's mental health has profound effects on individuals, communities, and economies.	Direct	Effective	[49]
7	Traffic may cause physical disturbances, mental illness, and reduced social interaction.	Direct	Effective	[17]

(continued)

Table 7.4 (continued)

Relationship	Item	Direction of relationship	How the relationship is?	Reference
8	Upbringing and social changes within the city can interact with genetic risk factors and cause the development and exacerbation of mental illnesses, including stress and anxiety.	Direct	They interact	[2]
9	Living in neighborhoods with higher private car density, due to chronic noise, is associated with more stress symptoms.	Direct	Effective	[16]
10	Better urban planning in the field of urban mental health would make it possible to save about 1.2 trillion dollars yearly worldwide.	Direct	Effective	[9]
11	Traffic may cause physical disturbances, mental illness, and reduced social interaction.	Direct	Effective	[17]
12	Neighborhood form and social environment are related.	Direct	Being related	[16]
13	The longer and more complicated daily routes, and the more monofunctional the destinations, the more stressful a person experiences.	Direct	They interact	[8]
14	The problems faced by the urban poor have many psychological and social effects, leading to urban stress.	Direct	Effective	[50]
15	Living in deprived areas of the city, regardless of the individual's socio-economic status, is associated with behavioral and psychological problems in children.	Indirect	Effective	[51]
16	The characteristics of an urban environment (such as disorderly architecture, advertising, traffic, noise, etc.) can promote cognitive deficits.	Direct	Effective	[22]

Table 7.4 (continued)

Relationship	Item	Direction of relationship	How the relationship is?	Reference
17	The characteristics of an urban environment (such as disorderly architecture, advertising, traffic, noise, etc.) can promote cognitive deficits.	Indirect	Effective	[22]
18	Land uses have environmental (climate changes, the extent of pollutants, etc.), social (demographic changes, security changes), and economic (employment, unemployment, poverty, income, and spatial justice) consequences.	Direct	Effective	[26]
19	Land uses have environmental (climate changes, the extent of pollutants, etc.), social (demographic changes, security changes), and economic (employment, unemployment, poverty, income, and spatial justice) consequences.	Direct	Effective	[26]
20	Land uses have environmental (climate changes, the extent of pollutants, etc.), social (demographic changes, security changes), and economic (employment, unemployment, poverty, income, and spatial justice) consequences.	Direct	Effective	[26]
21	The commercialization of main walls affects the spatial quality of residential areas.	Direct	Effective	[26]
22	Land uses can cause spatial–physical deterioration.	Direct	Effective	[26]
23	Cultural differences, citizens' fear of the stigma associated with mental illness and insufficient insurance coverage, etc., can cause the non-use of mental health services.	Direct	Effective	[40]

(continued)

Table 7.4 (continued)

Relationship	Item	Direction of relationship	How the relationship is?	Reference
24	Residential stability of the neighborhood and the concentration of the elderly, regardless of indicators of economic deprivation, is an aspect of social integration.	Direct	They interact	[16]
	The starter house policy, if properly implemented, will lead to more stable housing, better community integration, and a higher quality of life for homeless people with severe mental illness. Of course, patients who suffer from paranoia will be usually not comfortable in group housing.	Direct	Effective	[22]
25	Targeted social services reduce the effects of poverty, migration, and homelessness.	Direct	Effective	[21]

- Educational opportunities affect the degree of perceived respect for the community through their impact on social capital.

The number of such relationships in Fig. 7.2 is very large and only a few of them are stated in this section. Table 7.3 presents information about the relationships shown in the figure and the references from which they were extracted. First, the intended text is specified in the form of the item and then, the content of the extracted relationships is stated.

7.6 Examining the Relationship Between Stress-Relief Urban Planning Dimensions

How the dimensions of stress-relief urban planning interact with each other is very important. For this purpose, after examining the relationships between the effective indicators in this section using the (Maxqda) software, the relationships between the dimensions abovementioned were examined in the theoretical research framework in the form of Fig. 7.3. It should be noted that the references and how these dimensions are related are presented in Table 7.4.

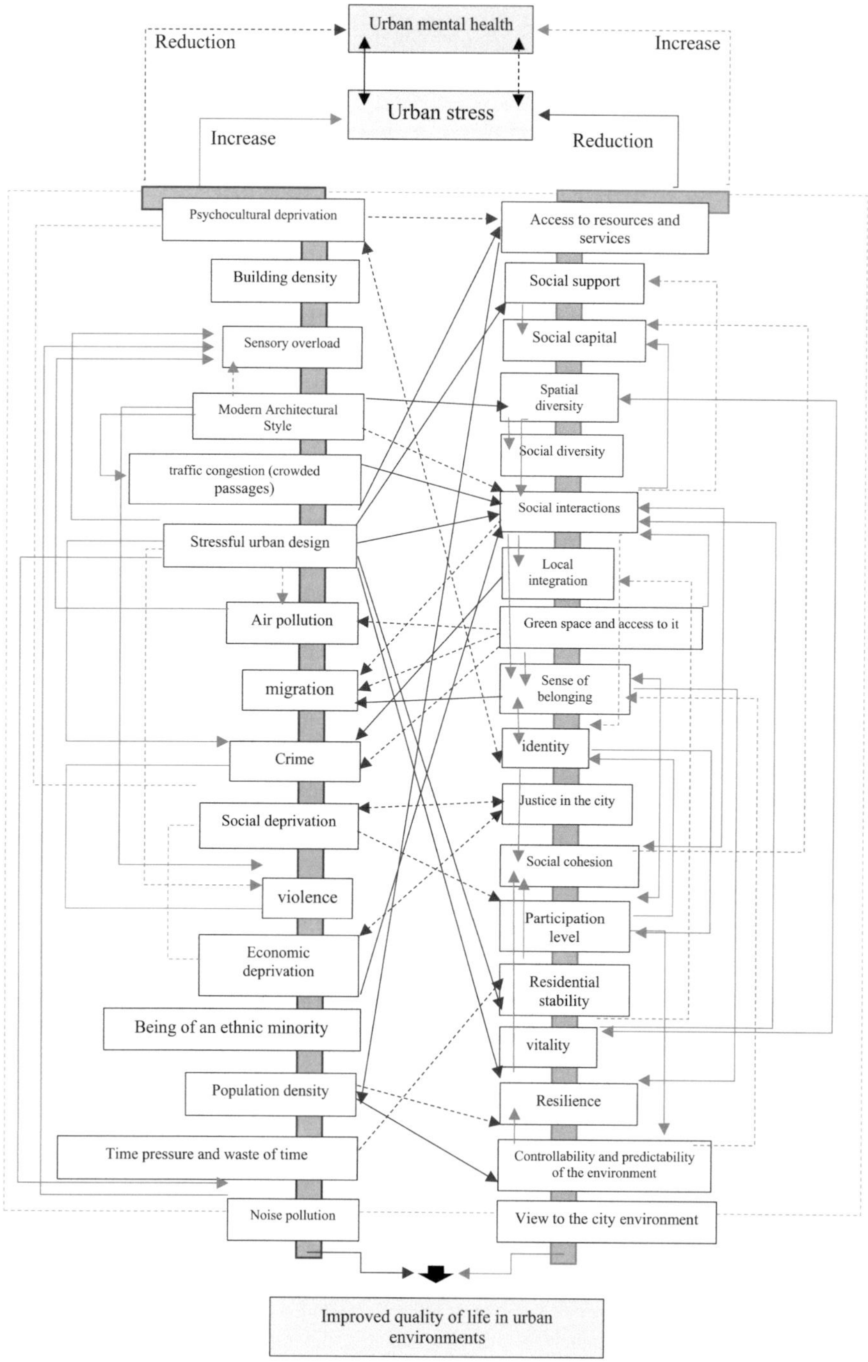

Fig. 7.4 The conceptual model

7.7 Conclusion and Presentation of the Conceptual Model

In this section, after identifying the relationship between urban mental health and urban stress in Fig. 4.2, the general research indicators are presented in the form of the theoretical framework and Fig. 7.1 and the relationships between them are shown in Fig. 7.2. Moreover, according to the relationships presented in the previous sections and the most important and influential general research indicators, the research conceptual model is presented in Fig. 7.4. According to this figure, urban mental health and urban stress mutually influence each other (directly and indirectly). The indicators extracted from theoretical foundations are classified into two groups. The first group increases urban stress and consequently reduces urban mental health, and the second group reduces urban stress and consequently improves mental health. It should be noted that in the presented conceptual model, relationships in blue indicate an increase, and relationships in red indicate a decrease. Finally, after examining the final effects and consequences of stress-relief urban planning, the quality of life in urban environments has been identified as the most important and comprehensive effect of this planning.

References

1. Lyn E, Daniel F, Garety PA. The psychological effect of an urban environment on individuals with persecutory delusions: the Camberwell walk study. Schizophr Res. 2008;99(1–3):77–84. https://doi.org/10.1016/j.schres.2007.10.027.
2. Pykett J, Osborne T, Resch B. From urban stress to neurourbanism: how should we research city well-being? Ann Am Assoc Geogr. 2020;2020:1–16. https://doi.org/10.1080/24694452.2020.1736982.
3. Buttazzoni A, Doherty S, Minaker L. How do urban environments affect young people's mental health? A novel conceptual framework to bridge public health, planning, and neurourbanism. Public Health Rep. 2021;137:48–61. https://doi.org/10.1177/0033354920982088.
4. Coope J, Barrett A, Brown B, Crossley M, Raghavan R, Sivakami M. Resilience, mental health and urban migrants: a narrative review. Int J Migr Health Soc Care. 2020;16(2):137–59. https://doi.org/10.1108/ijmhsc-04-2019-0048.
5. Adli M, Schondorf J. Macht uns die Stadt krank. Wirkung von Stadtstress auf Emotionen, Verhalten und psychische Gesundheit; Does the city make us ill? The effect of urban stress on emotions, behavior, and mental health. Bundesgesundheitsbl. 2020;63:979–86. https://doi.org/10.1007/s00103-020-03185-w.
6. Mubi Brighenti A, Pavoni A. City of unpleasant feelings. Stress, comfort and animosity in urban life. Soc Cult Geogr. 2017;20:1–20. https://doi.org/10.1080/14649365.2017.1355065.
7. Sigmund B, Mijatovic M. Gesundheit in der Stadt. 2019. https://www.detail.de. Accessed 22 Sept 2021.
8. Adli M, Berger M, Brakemeier E-L, Engel L, Fingerhut J, Hehl R, et al. Neurourbanistik – ein methodischer Schulterschluss zwischen Stadtplanung und Neurowissenschaften. Die Psychiatrie. 2016;13:70–8.
9. D'Acci LS. Urbanicity mental costs valuation: a review and urban-societal planning consideration. Mind Soc. 2020;9:223–35. https://doi.org/10.1007/s11299-020-00235-3.
10. Lewis CA, Sturgill S. Comment: Healing in the urban environment a person/plant viewpoint. J Am Plan Assoc. 1979;45(3):330–8. https://doi.org/10.1080/01944367908976971.

11. Gruebner O, Rapp MA, Adli M, Kluge U, Galea S, Heinz A. Cities and mental health. Dtsch Arztebl Int. 2017;114:121–7. https://doi.org/10.3238/arztebl.2017.0121.
12. Knöll M, Neuheuser K, Cleff T, Rudolph-Cleff A. A tool to predict perceived urban stress in open public spaces. Environ Plan B Urban Anal City Sci. 2017;45:797–813. https://doi.org/10.1177/0265813516686971.
13. Miller KM, Phillips MH. Correlates of urban stress and mental health: the impact of social context on resilience. J Soc Distress Homeless. 2005;14(1–2):46–64. https://doi.org/10.1179/105307805807066301.
14. Manning N. Sociology, biology and mechanisms in urban mental health. Soc Theory Health. 2018;17:1–22. https://doi.org/10.1057/s41285-018-00085-7.
15. Joshua CF, Freeman C, Bazargan-Hejazi S. Environmental interventions for physical and mental health: challenges and opportunities for Greater Los Angeles. Int J Environ Res Public Health. 2019;16(12):2180. https://doi.org/10.3390/ijerph16122180.
16. Miles R, Coutts C, Mohamadi A. Neighborhood urban form, social environment, and depression. J Urban Health. 2012;89(1):1–18. https://doi.org/10.1007/s11524-011-9621-2.
17. Rishi P, Khuntia G. Urban environmental stress and behavioral adaptation in Bhopal City of India. Urban Stud Res. 2012;2012:1–9. https://doi.org/10.1155/2012/635061.
18. Li J, Rose N. Urban social exclusion and mental health of China's rural-urban migrants – a review and call for research. Health Place. 2017;48:20–30. https://doi.org/10.1016/j.healthplace.2017.08.009.
19. Okkels N, Kristiansen CB, Munk-Jørgensen P, Sartorius N. Urban mental health. Curr Opin Psychiatry. 2018;31:258–64. https://doi.org/10.1097/YCO.0000000000000413.
20. Larcombe E, Logan P, Horwitz A. High-rise apartments and urban mental health—historical and contemporary views. Challenges. 2019;10(2):34. https://doi.org/10.3390/challe10020034.
21. Ventriglio A, Torales J, Castaldelli-Maia JM, De Berardis D, Bhugra D. Urbanization and emerging mental health issues. CNS Spectr. 2020;2020:1–8. https://doi.org/10.1017/S1092852920001236.
22. Baumann PS, Söderström O, Abrahamyan Empson L, Söderström D, Codeluppi Z, Golay P, et al. Urban remediation: a new recovery-oriented strategy to manage urban stress after first-episode psychosis. Soc Psychiatry Psychiatr Epidemiol. 2019;55:273–83. https://doi.org/10.1007/s00127-019-01795-7.
23. Haines MM, Stansfeld SA, Job RFS, Berglund B, Head J. Chronic aircraft noise exposure, stress responses, mental health and cognitive performance in school children. Psychol Med. 2001;31(2):265–77. https://doi.org/10.1017/S0033291701003282.
24. Seth P, Murray CC, Braxton ND, DiClemente RJ. The concrete jungle: city stress and substance abuse among young adult African American men. J Urban Health. 2012;90(2):307–13. https://doi.org/10.1007/s11524-012-9716-4.
25. Meloni A, Fornara F, Carrus G. Predicting pro-environmental behaviors in the urban context: the direct or moderated effect of urban stress, city identity, and worldviews. Cities. 2019;88:83–90. https://doi.org/10.1016/j.cities.2019.01.001.
26. Forouhar A, Kheyroddin R. The impact of commercialization on the spatial quality of residential neighbourhoods: evidence from Nasr neighbourhood of Tehran. Geogr Plann Space. 2016;6:63–84.
27. Nnebue CC, Adinma ED, Queencallista N. Urbanization and health. Orient J Med. 2014;26:1–2.
28. Franz G, Wiener JM. From space syntax to space semantics: a behaviorally and perceptually oriented methodology for the efficient description of the geometry and topology of environments. Environ Plann B Plann Des. 2008;35(4):574–92. https://doi.org/10.1068/b33050.
29. Scheydt S, Müller Staub M, Frauenfelder F, Nielsen GH, Behrens J, Needham I. Sensory overload: a concept analysis. Int J Ment Health Nurs. 2017;26(2):110–20. https://doi.org/10.1111/inm.12303.
30. Young J. Personal knowledge capital. In: Social capital and trust for a web environment; 2012. p. 81–90. https://doi.org/10.1016/b978-1-84334-700-2.50007-5.

31. Shirkhani M, Vaseiezadeh NS. Social capital and economic development: a comparative study of Iran and South Korea. Polit Q. 2011;41(2):213–32. Persian.
32. Schwarzer C. Encyclopedia of applied psychology. Soc Support. 2004;2004:435–41. https://doi.org/10.1016/b0-12-657410-3/00414-1.
33. Taylor PJ, Gooding P, Wood AM, Tarrier N. The role of defeat and entrapment in depression, anxiety, and suicide. Psychol Bull. 2011;137(3):391–420. https://doi.org/10.1037/a0022935.
34. Allen B. Culture of social sciences. Translated by Sarokhani B. Tehran: Kayhan Publications; 1996. Persian.
35. Ebadollahi H, Piri A, Movaghar Narbin M. Stigma and social identity: the case of individuals with visible physical disabilities in Rasht. Soc Probl Iran. 2012;2:195–222. Persian.
36. Thorns, David C. The transformation of cities: urban theory and urban life. 2002. https://doi.org/10.1007/978-1-4039-9031-0.
37. Amiri M, Vedadhir A. Stigma and discrimination: two vital social oppressions influencing on disclosure of HIV status by patients with HIV/AIDS. Soc Probl Iran. 2018;8:1–23. Persian. https://doi.org/10.22059/ijsp.2018.65051.
38. Chalabi M, Amir Kafi M. Multilevel analysis of social isolation. Iran J Soc. 2004;5:3–31. Persian.
39. Jevtic M. Building capacity for public urban mental health – example of Reflecting Citizens workshops. Eur J Pub Health. 2020;30:ckaa165.975. https://doi.org/10.1093/eurpub/ckaa165.975.
40. Caracci G. Urban mental health: an international survey. Int J Ment Health. 2006;35(1):39–45. https://doi.org/10.2753/imh0020-7411350103.
41. Alcock I, White MP, Wheeler BW, Fleming LE, Depledge MH. Longitudinal effects on mental health of moving to greener and less green urban areas. Environ Sci Technol. 2014;48(2):1247–55. https://doi.org/10.1021/es403688w.
42. Galea S, Freudenberg N, Vlahov D. Cities and population health. Soc Sci Med. 2005;60(5):1017–33.
43. Saberifar R. Investigate the relationship between urban furniture and utilization of urban spaces with mental health. Health Res J. 2018;3:89–94. https://doi.org/10.29252/hrjbaq.3.2.89.
44. Amari H. Psychology, city and daily life. Tehran: Tisa Publications; 2014.
45. Mirzaei M, Movahed K. The effect of color of medical buildings in reducing stress and length of treatment (Case study: Kowsar Hospital, Shiraz). J Urban Dev Architect Environ Identity. 2020;1(3):60–72. https://doi.org/10.22034/(jrupa-ei).2020.120233.
46. Burton I. Factors in urban stress. J Sociol Soc Welf. 1990;17(1).
47. Elsamahy EM, Abd El-Fattah R. Designing non-stressed psychological public spaces. BAU J Health Wellbeing. 2018;2018:121–32.
48. Capineri C, Huang H, Gartner G. Tracking emotions in urban space. Two experiments in Vienna and Siena. Riv Geogr Ital. 2018;125(2):273–88.
49. Lloyd S, Kelly R, Kimberly G, Joshua R. Challenges of urban mental health disaster planning. J Aggress Maltreat Trauma. 2005;10(3):695–706. https://doi.org/10.1300/J146v10n03_03.
50. Ewart CK, Suchday S. Discovering how urban poverty and violence affect health: development and validation of a neighborhood stress index. Health Psychol. 2002;21(3):254–62. https://doi.org/10.1037/0278-6133.21.3.254.
51. Kalff AC, Kroes M, Vles JS, Hendriksen JG, Feron FJ, Steyaert J, et al. Neighbourhood level and individual level SES effects on child problem behaviour: a multilevel analysis. J Epidemiol Commun Health. 2001;55(4):246–50. https://doi.org/10.1136/jech.55.4.246.

Chapter 8
Conclusion

Abstract In this chapter, the findings of the previous chapters are explained first, and then the findings of this book are compared with previous research. Finally, the opportunities for future research and the conclusion are presented. Stress-relief urban planning, as planning closely related to urban mental health and improving the quality of urban life, is very important in this century. In fact, the findings of this book reveal that urban mental health and urban stress have direct and indirect mutual effects on each other. Also, the level of urban stress can be evaluated by the indicators identified in the dimensions of use and activity, physical form, transportation, environmental, social, economic, cultural, housing, and individual traits. The indicators extracted from theoretical studies are classified into two groups: (a) indicators that increase urban stress and reduce urban mental health, including psycho-cultural deprivation, building density, sensory overload, modern architectural style, traffic density, stressful urban design, crowding, air pollution, immigration, crime, social deprivation, violence, economic deprivation, ethnic minority, population density, time pressure and waste of time, and noise pollution; and (b) indicators that reduce urban stress and increase urban mental health, including access to resources and services, social support, social capital, spatial diversity, social diversity, social interactions, local integration, green space and access to it, sense of belonging, identity, justice in the city, social cohesion, participation rate, urban sustainability, vitality, resilience, controllability and predictability of the environment, and view of the city environment up to 10 m.

Keywords Urban stress · Stress-relief urban planning · Mental health

8.1 Introduction

In this chapter, the findings of the previous chapters are explained first, and then the findings of this book are compared with previous research. Finally, the opportunities for future research and the conclusion are presented.

S. Jalilisadrabad et al., *Stress Relief Urban Planning*,
https://doi.org/10.1007/978-981-99-4202-2_8

8.2 Research Findings

In this section, the research findings are presented as follows:

- Explaining concepts such as health, mental health, urban health, stress, environmental stress, and urban stress.
- Explaining the relationship between city, mental health, and urban stress using content analysis technique and (Maxqda) software.
- Explaining the factors causing urban environments stressful and their repetition and importance using categorical content analysis and (Maxqda) software.
- Identifying effective solutions to improve mental comfort and reduce stress in urban environments.
- Identifying urban stress measurement methods and introducing the best method.
- Investigating the research background in the form of two parts of the international background and the domestic background.
- Examining global experiences and summarizing the solutions and indicators presented in them using content analysis.
- Introducing stress-relief urban planning and its characteristics.
- Presenting the theoretical framework and general indicators of stress-relief urban planning according to urban stressors and global experiences.
- Examining the relationships between stress-relief urban planning indicators using content analysis technique and (Maxqda) software.
- Examining the relationships between the stress-relief urban planning dimensions using content analysis technique and (Maxqda) software.
- Presenting the conceptual model of stress-relief urban planning after determining the relationships between indicators and identifying the most important and influential general indicators.

8.3 Comparison of the Findings of This Research with Those of Previous Research

Considering Sect. 8.2, this section compares the findings of this research with those of previous research. The review of the research background shows that many studies have been carried out in the field of urban mental health applying different approaches. Reviewing the urban mental health literature indicates seven approaches: (1) exploratory studies that lead to the discovery of the relationship between urbanization and mental health, (2) library studies that attempt to summarize and organize theoretical foundations, (3) comparative studies that compare places, some of which are listed in Table 2.1, (4) detailed studies that address a specific problem or mental illness in cities, such as stress, depression, schizophrenia, etc., or the effects of mental health on a specific part of the city, such as housing, (5) studies that identify factors affecting urban mental health, (6) studies that provide specific guidelines influencing the subject, and (7) studies that are not included in the abovementioned six categories.

The research background of urban stress also shows that The study of urban stress started with Simmel's [1] classic thesis. He considered the modern city as an inevitable psychologically stimulating environment and in the late nineteenth century, he proposed factors such as sensitivity to noise and air pollution. Simmel sought to develop two sciences: the analysis of urban effects (as the science of psychic stimulation and the measurement of its effects) and the analysis of urban rhythms (as the science of individual brain stimulation) [1]. In the 1950s and 1960s, while Simmel's ideas were developing, Prindle recognized urban stress as the current disease of cities and considered it a disease caused by overcrowding, the most effective solution of which is to identify possible sources [2]. Next, Milgram [3] proposed the perspective of stimulus overload and adaptation strategies, analogized the city to the frozen world, and introduced the concept of familiar strangers [3]. Christmas [4] discussed the necessity of developing health services according to environmental stress [4]. Then, Lazarus and Cohen [5] emphasized the importance of studying environmental stress in real conditions and considered the laboratory inappropriate for this research [5]. Also, Burton [6] emphasized the necessity of longitudinal studies in this field [6]. Considering the approved relationship between urbanization and mental health by Faris and Dunham and the approved relationship between urbanization and stress by Simmel, this effect was proven by Lederbogen et al. [7] in a laboratory ambiance using brain imaging [7]. In 2016, the term "neuro urbanism" was proposed for the first time as a solution to urban stress, which resulted in the "Charta of Neurourbanism" in 2019 [8].

Since the beginning of the twentieth century, many studies have investigated the relationship between urbanization and stress and provided effective solutions to it with different approaches. However, no study has been carried out to develop stress-relief urban planning so far. Most studies have examined only part of the subject and have provided effective solutions in the same subject. The indicators and dimensions of this planning are not known comprehensively. Also, how the city is related to stress, effective solutions, and urban stress assessment methods have not been well studied.

8.4 Conclusion

The results of this research indicate that the city both directly influences mental health and causes stress through social, economic, physical, environmental, housing, transportation, and individual stressors, and this stress reduces mental health. Of course, because physical and mental health are highly interrelated, the city also affects mental health by degrading general or physical health. The city is also impacted by mental health, both directly and indirectly through stress and public health. Therefore, the effects of urbanisation on mental health as well as the effects of mental health on the city might be mediated by urban stress and physical health.

To make the most of urban life, it will be extremely helpful to have a greater understanding of this link, the role of mediators, and efforts to lessen the detrimental effects of cities on mental health.

The city's inhabitants are subjected to a lot of stressors, and this exposure is what leads to the development of mental illnesses in them. Despite the significance of both urban stress and mental health, there hasn't been enough study done on urban stressors, useful indicators, treatments, etc., or on the possible connections between built environment features and mental health. While it is crucial to pay attention to the aspects of the urban environment that affect mental health and stress, work to lessen these effects, and create urban planning and design that relieves stress.

The experts in this field consider urban stress to be mostly caused by social stressors and environmental stressors, followed by economic stressors, stressors associated with the physical form, transportation, land use and activity, housing, cultural stressors, and individual stressors, respectively. In fact, according to the experts in this field, social and environmental factors cause high stress in cities compared to villages. Of course, other factors are also very important and policymakers, planners, designers, and architects should take steps to reduce these stressors in the urban environment after understanding them properly.

According to the abovementioned, stress-relief urban planning, as planning closely related to urban mental health and improving the quality of urban life, is very important in this century. The findings of this book reveal that urban mental health and urban stress have direct and indirect mutual effects on each other. Also, the level of urban stress can be evaluated by the indicators identified in the dimensions of use and activity, physical form, transportation, environmental, social, economic, cultural, housing, and individual traits. The indicators extracted from theoretical studies are classified into two groups: (a) indicators that increase urban stress and reduce urban mental health, including psycho-cultural deprivation, building density, sensory overload, modern architectural style, traffic density, stressful urban design, crowding, air pollution, immigration, crime, social deprivation, violence, economic deprivation, ethnic minority, population density, time pressure and waste of time, and noise pollution; and (b) indicators that reduce urban stress and increase urban mental health, including access to resources and services, social support, social capital, spatial diversity, social diversity, social interactions, local integration, green space and access to it, sense of belonging, identity, justice in the city, social cohesion, participation rate, urban sustainability, vitality, resilience, controllability and predictability of the environment, and view of the city environment up to 10 m. Finally, after acquiring knowledge from the theoretical foundations and reviewing most of the published research in this field, the opportunities for future research are introduced as follows:

- Conducting longitudinal studies and analyzing the relationship between the duration of exposure to the city and mental health.
- Enhancing information about coping resources of the neighborhood and their effects on mental health and urban stress.
- Assessing the effects of each coping resource on the mental health of citizens.

- Investigating how to distribute urban resources in a more equitable, sustainable, and balanced way to reduce stress and promote mental health.
- Investigating how to reduce issues such as discrimination and social isolation and their effects.
- Identifying interventions that reduce urban stress in developing countries.
- Conducting interdisciplinary research between architecture, urban planning, epidemiology, geography, neuroscience, medicine, and sociology.
- Evaluating the effects of types of the built environment on psychological well-being through field studies.
- Examining the relationship between urban spaces and the psychological or biological behavior of people.
- Comprehensively identifying factors reducing urban stressors.
- Investigating the impact of urban design and planning on the processes of social, psychological, and emotional maturity of people.
- Identifying the scope of comprehensive mental health improvement plans in cities and how to develop, implement, and monitor them.
- Practically implementing stress-relief urban planning in cities and investigating its effects.

References

1. Simmel J. The metropolis and mental life. Section 7 of the people, place, and space reader, 1903, p. 223–6.
2. Prindle RA. Health aspects of the urban environment. Public Health Rep (1896–1970). 1968;83(7):617–21. https://doi.org/10.2307/4593367.
3. Milgram S. The experience of living in cities. Science. 1970;167(3924):1461–8. https://doi.org/10.1126/science.167.3924.1461.
4. Christmas JJ. Psychological stresses of urban living: new direction for mental health services in the inner city. J Natl Med Assoc. 1973;65(6):483–6, passim.
5. Lazarus RS, Cohen JB. Environmental stress. Hum Behav Environ. 1977;1977:89–127. https://doi.org/10.1007/978-1-4684-0808-9_3.
6. Burton I. Factors in urban stress. J Sociol Soc Welf. 1990;17(1).
7. Lederbogen F, Kirsch P, Haddad L, Streit F, Tost H, Schuch P, et al. City living and urban upbringing affect neural social stress processing in humans. Nature. 2011;474:498–501.
8. Adli M, Berger M, Brakemeier E-L, Engel L, Fingerhut J, Hehl R, et al. Neurourbanistik – ein methodischer Schulterschluss zwischen Stadtplanung und Neurowissenschaften. Die Psychiatrie. 2016;13:70–8.

MIX
Papier aus verantwortungsvollen Quellen
Paper from responsible sources
FSC® C105338

If you have any concerns about our products,
you can contact us on
ProductSafety@springernature.com

In case Publisher is established outside the EU,
the EU authorized representative is:
Springer Nature Customer Service Center GmbH
Europaplatz 3, 69115 Heidelberg, Germany

Printed by Libri Plureos GmbH
in Hamburg, Germany